SELF-ACTUATED

HEALING

BY LONNY J. BROWN, PH.D.

"They're healing warts with hypnosis, high blood pressure with biofeedback, cancer with visualization, colitis with relaxation, arthritis with yoga, headaches with meditation."

New Age Magazine, *May, 1979*

LIBRARY OF CONGRESS CATALOGING IN PUBLICATION DATA

Books for a better world

NATUREGRAPH PUBLISHERS, INC.
P.O. Box 1075
Happy Camp, CA 96039
U.S.A.

Dedicated to my parents, Seymour and Birdie Brown,
who gave me life and love.

ACKNOWLEDGEMENTS

I wish to acknowledge my incalculable debts to the Great Teachers, whose wisdom and compassion have touched my life: Neem Karoli Baba, Rama Krishna, Paramahansa Yogananda, H.H. The Fourteenth Dalai Lama, H.H. The Sixteenth Karmapa, Chogyam Trungpa Rimpoche, Lama Kalu Rimpoche, Alan Watts, Kahlil Gibran, Rudolph Steiner, and many more of the Lights among us. And of course, how can one thank The Buddha and Christ?

I express my deepest gratitude to my Dharma friends, who have helped me to see a bit more clearly: Ram Dass, Tsultrim Allione, Katherine Usha, Bhagwan Dass, Joseph Goldstein, Jack Kornfield, and Dr. Robert Hover.

I am also very thankful for the help and support of Dr. Barbara DuBois, Chris Sarfaty, Dr. Geri Brooks, Peter Johnson, Anita Francis, and Dawn June.

Finally, I must thank the following generous souls who, over the years of fantasy and frustration, gave me the ultimate vote of confidence—money!: Sy and Birdie, Mrs. June Silverberg, Sindy and Mark Levine, Sue Bonner, Perry Garfinkle and Iris, Peter Gannett, Cecil and Elsie Lyon, Fred and Justine Eaton, Mrs. Lilla Rose Levitt, Edith Spenser, Sheila Simon, The New Hampshire Charitable Fund, Goddard College, and Columbia Pacific University.
God bless you all!

Lonny J. Brown
New Hampshire,
July, 1987

Kostoglotov (said) "We shouldn't behave like rabbits and put our complete trust in doctors. For instance, I'm reading this book." He picked up a large, open book from the window sill. "Abrikosov and Stryukov, Pathological Anatomy, medical school textbook. It says here that the link between the development of tumors and the central nervous system has so far been very little studied. And this link is an amazing thing! It's written here in so many words." He found the place. " 'It happens rarely, but there are cases of self-induced healing.' You see how it's worded? Not recovery through treatment, but actual healing! See?"

There was a stir throughout the ward. It was as though "self-induced healing" had fluttered out of the great open book like a rainbow-colored butterfly for everyone to see, and they all held up their foreheads and cheeks for its healing touch as it flew past.

"Self-induced" said Kostoglotov, laying aside his book. He waved his hands, fingers splayed. "That means that suddenly for some unexplained reason the tumor starts off in the opposite direction! It gets smaller, resolves and finally disappears! See?"

They were all silent, gaping at the fairy tale. That a tumor, one's own tumor, the destructive tumor which had mangled one's whole life, should suddenly drain away, dry up and die by itself?

They were all silent, still holding their faces up to the butterfly. It was only the gloomy Podduyev who made his bed creak and, with a hopeless and obstinate expression on his face, croaked out, "I suppose for that you need to have ... a clear conscience."

—Alexander Solzhenitsyn: Cancer Ward

CONTENTS

◡◠◡◠◡◠

INTRODUCTION

The best way to live a long life is to get a serious ailment and take care of it.
                                                              —*Sir Wm. Osler*

This book is about you. The Real You. When you were born, you were an expression of organic perfection, or pretty near to it. Miraculously, you grew your bones and organs and brain, according to a billion-year-old living blueprint that you carry within. Some wise force, some unfailing energy made your heart beat and your breath flow, without trying. Physically you were the crowning achievement of natural evolution, the most astounding product of a marvelous universe.

Most likely, your perfect little body worked flawlessly. And it developed and repaired itself automatically. With a bit of luck, our body's innate health maintenance and repair mechanisms continue to function smoothly, involuntarily, into adulthood, and we enjoy normal health, in spite of the hazards of life. But sooner or later pain and *dis-ease* upsets this happy state, and we naturally look about for sources of relief.

Until recently (as western medical history goes), our search for cures has been through the hard sciences: primarily biology and chemistry. It was a highly externalized and material quest, with some remarkable gains made in the form of antibiotics, vaccines, and a large arsenal of chemically specific remedies which stimulate and regulate human metabolism. Today the very word medicine is taken as synonymous with "drug."

The problem is that after conquering the infectious diseases, we tried to apply *material* medicine to our more modern, *immaterial* sicknesses—the diseases of civilization; of stress, and pollution; of nutritional deficiencies, and debilitating behaviors. The search continued to be focused in the test tube, while it should have been in the patients. Even Louis Pasteur repudiated the completeness of his contagion theory of disease, when he realized that susceptibility is variable. Germs weren't the only factor.

Only recently has it been recognized by science (and therefore the mass media) that non-physical factors—belief, motivation, emotions, the mind, the "heart"—play a vital role in both illness and recovery. In the East this has been known for ages, and the internal sciences of self-regulation and self-development became as highly perfected there as our external, "hard" sciences are in the West. We have much to learn from the oriental healing arts, as well as a thing or two to teach them. Just as the arrival of vaccinations against smallpox signaled new hope in India, so too the appearance of meditation classes in western hospitals offers a sign of hope in our "stressed out" society. It is encouraging to witness, and exciting to participate in this great integration of health sciences, the internal and external, East and West.

But, ironically, for all the resources spent on medicine and health care, remarkably few people really seem interested in learning how to actually get themselves well. If and when enough sick people want to take charge of their health, our hospitals will also become schools for self-healing. Until then, don't expect your doctor to tell you how to heal yourself, unless she or he has both the philosophy and tools to address your whole being. The best of the new breed of holistic health practitioners are part doctor, part minister, and part teacher, yet they merely act as catalysts to one's own self-discovery.

This book is for those who are ready to get on with it. Its

premise is simple: that very same essential, indwelling intelligence that grew your perfect baby body, that oxidizes and metabolizes nutrients, that learns to recognize and fight harmful micro-organisms, that daily controls and transforms trillions of cells into a network of wise, living tissue—that central power of your being, by which you live and breathe and have your existence—is waiting to be utilized for self healing. You can obstruct it, cooperate with it, or more importantly, you can enhance your body's own healing capacities. Rather than wait and hope for health, you can optimize the process with intelligent self-care strategies that are effective, rewarding, and risk free. Not only does conscious participation in healing make for quicker, more successful, and complete recovery, but as we shall see, in some cases, it even makes the difference between health and irreversible decline.

Self-actuated healing can only come from within. A drug or treatment, even an idea, might activate you, but only you can *actuate* you! The word implies origin of being, and conscious choice. Health and longevity are not accidents. Sometime after youth, you have to get intentional about it. The good news is that you can *learn* how to generate energy, repair your parts, balance your systems, preserve your faculties, and renew your life.

Realizing the possibilities is a first important step. If, through inspiration, guidance, motivation, and practice, you can awaken to your own true nature—your Whole Self—then you will understand Self-Actuated Healing. In the hope of facilitating that most valuable realization, I offer the information that follows.

~~~~~~

MY MIRACULOUS BODY

- The combined pulling strength of all the muscles in my body equals 25 tons.
- My heart pumps the equivalent of five to six thousand quarts of blood through me every day.
- There are more bacteria living on and in my body than there are people on the earth. Most of them are benign and even beneficial: I depend on intestinal bacteria to help me digest my food.
- My body secretes more than seven quarts of digestive juices daily.
- My ears can discriminate among more than 300,000 tones. Factory noise is one million times as loud as a soft whisper.
- My brain, many times more complex than the most advanced computers, operates on the amount of electrical power that would light a 10-watt bulb.
- My eyes can distinguish nearly eight million differences in colors.
- The surface area of my lungs is 1,000 square feet—20 times greater than the surface area of my skin.
- My bones manufacture one billion new red blood cells every day, replacing old ones at the rate of two and one-half million per second.
- My blood serum is almost identical in chemical content to sea water.
- My circulatory system is more than 70 thousand miles long.
- Every pound of excess fat I carry requires an extra 200 miles of capillaries.
- My digestive tract is 30 feet long.
- One cubic inch of my bone can withstand a two-ton force.

~~~~~~

∽∾∿∾∽∾∿

I.

THE HEALING MIND

Insofar as we see health as the victorious outcome of a war of annihilation against germs, viruses, tumors and other invaders, we are likely to overlook the role played by our own habits, thinking patterns and belief structures... Non-physical agents like relationships with a mother-in-law or unsympathetic boss, or financial difficulties can produce pathologic tissue change. Thoughts of helplessness and defeat impede the flow of air to the lungs, just as frustration and rage block the flow of blood to the heart. Thoughts, like germs and poison, can induce disease.

Irving Oyle
The New American Medical Show

Modern psycho-biology and psychosomatic medicine have made important progress in recent years in verifying, if not completely understanding, the link between mind and body in the cause of disease. We now accept that chronic anxiety can lead to ulcers; that unacknowledged fears can cause headaches, and that mental depression also depresses the immune system.[1] We have come to recognize the psychological profiles behind the businessman's ulcer, the cancer-prone personality[2] and coronary high-risk "Type A Behavior"[3]. Clearly, the mind plays a key role in the origins of many illnesses. Indeed, one of the insights of holism as a new paradigm in medicine is the inter-active, inter-dependent nature of the complete organism, physical to mental to spiritual, dense to subtle, material to energetic.

The current challenge in medicine is to explore and exploit this vital relationship between psyche and soma for purposes of healing (and ultimately for prevention as well). *If we can make ourselves sick with grief, fear, anger, bad expectations, and other negative states of mind, we can also use positive mental states to get well.*

Self-healing involves personal psychological dynamics such as expectation, self-image, goals, imagination, will power, enthusiasm, faith, and the full range of possible mental, emotional, and spiritual states. The chapters that follow include clinical evidence, personal accounts, and expert testimony about the primacy of mind in all states of health and illness, plus an over-view of the major new techniques and strategies that utilize this mind/body connection in self-healing. Call it psycho-spiritual behavioral medicine.

Of course, this is not really a very new idea. The field of placebo research, for example, has been systematically investigating the role and power of the belief system in healing for at least 60 years.[4] In fact there is good indication that such medical luminaries of the past as Hippocrates and Sir William Osler were well aware of the crucial importance of the patient's expectations in determining the outcome of their interventions.

More recently, the pioneering works of the Simontons, Dr. Lawrence LeShan, Norman Cousins, Dr. Bernie Siegel and Dr. Herbert Benson have demonstrated the value of the new behavioral/transformational psychotherapies in cases of "terminal" cancer and other catastrophic illnesses. Today, consciousness-based therapies such as autogenic training, biofeedback, meditation and visualization have become, in many cases the treatments of choice, and the most risk-free interventions for migraine headaches, hypertension and circulatory disorders, chronic pain, and a variety of stress-related systemic disfunctions.

All of these methods radically shift the focus of attention

in healing from medicines to the mind. (Dr. Gerald Jampolsky
calls the holistic/spiritual approach he uses with children with
catastrophic illnesses *Attitudinal Healing.*[5]) The approach
operates within the intangible domain of the psyche, yet
demonstrates profound physical influence on organ function,
cell development, hormonal balance, circulation, muscle
tone, temperature, and other physiological indicators. Indeed,
no mental/emotional event takes place in thought, without a
corresponding change, subtle or gross, in the physical body.
As we shall see, the New Medicine is now able to capitalize
on this correspondency with the introduction of precise,
easily learned, mind-based, self-healing skills. Later chapters
discuss the therapeutic implications of relaxation, meditation, yoga and breathing exercises, among others.

   In recognizing the mutual interdependence of psychology and pathology, we are saying in effect that they are no
longer separate sciences. These developments point to the
resolution of the centuries-old mind/body dichotomy. The
Cartesian division is a false one. Bodymind is one unity.
Holism transcends both the spiritualist view—that man is
really a "higher" being somehow trapped within matter,
needing to escape—and the biological-materialist notion that
we are merely meat that just happens to generate thought, as
a kind of epi-phenomenon. Actually, at the neuro-synaptic
level, where electromagnetic nerve impulses, chemical
reactions, and thought all play out their parts in the perpetual
re-creation of conscious life, *none of them comes first.* We can
finally lay to rest the puzzle of causality when we realize the
virtual simultaneity, and the mutually interdependent, feed-
back-loop nature of body/mind/spirit processes. In other
words, we are whole ! The task is to *actualize* our realization of
this wholeness, and use it for self-healing.

MENTAL IMMUNITY

There is a direct connection between a robust will to live and the chemical balances in the brain. Creativity produces the vital brain impulses that stimulate the pituitary glands, triggering effects in the pineal glands and the whole of the endocrine system.

—Norman Cousins[6]

Norman Cousins, one of the more well known educators in behavioral medicine, likes to point out that the brain is the largest gland in the human body—a "natural apothecary." In the last decade, we have discovered endorphins, enkephalins, peptides, gamma globulin, interferon, norepinephrin and other mood- and sensitivity-mediating chemical "neuro-transmitters" in the brain. These neuro-humoral transducers are secreted selectively into the nervous system and blood supply in response to messages from the body, mind, and emotions. They profoundly influence both our experience and performance in the world. Usually released at times of emergency and stress, they may also be triggered by peak sports activities, religious experiences, and internal self-regulatory techniques such as yoga and meditation. Although present in the most minute quantities, these compounds are available in a vast number of possible combinations, and act as powerful regulators of our physical and mental sense of ourselves. They account for, among other things, the experience of "runner's high," and that thoroughly pleasant glow we feel after a good round of "belly laughter," or sex. For pain control they are virtually the body's own built-in morphine supply, called "opioids."

In a complex chemical balancing act within the brain, these potent substances also directly affect the efficiency of the immune system.[7] Through this brain/mind/body connection, we can now skillfully exploit the human mind's own potential influence over many formerly intractable systemic disorders. Cancer, arthritis, heart and blood diseases, and various glandular and organ disfunctions are proving responsive to mind-based therapies.[8]

But modern medicine has yet to fully appreciate or utilize

the great healing powers of the mind. This may be due to the scientific bias against employing anything that is not completely understood. Or it may be that recognizing the likes of visualization, hypnosis, and placebo as legitimate therapeutic tools would represent a threat to the medical establishment, the reputation of which has been built largely on the efficacy of the pharmacological (biochemical) approach to cure. Placebo research seriously calls into question the near-universal but relatively unexamined assumption that drugs "work" primarily by virtue of their chemical effects on the system, as opposed to their psychological impact within the Doctor/Patient healing relationship.* Indeed, this work threatens to vindicate Shamanism and other "superstitious" or "primitive" healing methods, a step which the medical mainstream is still quite reluctant to take.

Physicians have disregarded the tremendous potential of the mind (and "heart") in healing at the expense of their own effectiveness, and to the disadvantage of their patients, in several unforseen ways. Implicit in the possibility of the positive psychological influence of expectation on health is the equally significant negative influence: the *nocebo*. The classic example of this harmful disregard for the formidable power of suggestion is the insidious and often lethal effect of the terminal diagnosis on the highly suggestible patient with a life-threatening illness. In fact, one of the more potent influences on outcome for such cases is the relative degree of optimism or pessimism displayed by the doctor when giving the prognosis. Doctors' attitudes are contagious. When the message conveyed is strictly "bad news," and leaves little room for hope, the patient's belief system, and importantly, that of the family, is enlisted in the negative conspiracy to expect the worst; and because of the very real physical effects of such expectations, that's usually what they get.

A simple awareness of the importance of this crucial

---

* Hippocrates revealed his doubts when he wrote: "treat as many patients as possible with the new drugs while they still have the power to heal.

dynamic between doctor and patient at times of crisis could significantly alter the outcome in a favorable direction, in medically precarious cases. Norman Cousins recounts the following ideal scenario:

When (the Doctor) gets patients with new diagnoses of cancer, he sits down with them and tells them he's convinced they are going to make it. He tells them it's nonsense to equate the word "cancer" with death. He tells them he has an excellent treatment for their condition, and that they have an excellent treatment of their own— their body's own natural healing processes. "And you can activate that healing process," he tells them, "by building up your confidence in yourself and your confidence in me. By building up your joy, your appreciation of life, by your urge to go on to do everything you've wanted to do." He tells them that they're in possession of the most magical system the world has ever known for the treatment of disease.

"Now," he says, "here's the partnership I propose. I'll work with you on the things you'll be doing to build up your confidence, your joy, your hope, your faith. Beginning tomorrow, I'm going to introduce you to five other patients who had exactly the same kind of cancer you have and came through it successfully. I will make sure you receive the best treatment medical science has to offer. We're going to have a lot going for us, and I'm convinced that we can whip this thing and that you can make it." Then he holds out his hand and says, "Now how about a partnership?" They always take his hand.

Cousins goes on to describe another enlightened doctor's skillful communication with a patient with prostate cancer. A "CAT" scan showed that the cancer had spread throughout his body; they were able to identify 230 separate tumors:

The doctor sat down with the patient and said, "Well, Michael, I can't conceal from you the fact that this is very serious. You have cancer, and it's spreading. But serious as it is, I'm convinced that you can make it through. I've seen many cases, far more serious than your own, which have completely remitted. I think those cases have remitted because there's been a strong partnership between doctor and patient. I would like the two of us to join in such a partnership. My job will be to knock out the male hormone. I'm going to give you estrogen. We may also have to have some surgery. Your job is to have the best time of your life. I want you to exercise your will to live as you've never exercised it before. Vitamin C can help restore adrenal function, and the adrenal glands become depleted in many illnesses, so I think you should begin taking Vitamin C."

"I want you to eat the most highly nutritious diet you can possibly arrange, because I've got a hunch that many cancer patients die as much of malnutrition as they do of the disease itself. You've got to become extremely strong—through regular, gentle exercise. Strengthen your body in every possible way. If you do so, the treatments I'll be giving you will have a much better chance. I think you have a very good chance. I'm willing to do all I can from my end. Now, how about it!

This wise doctor succeeded in changing a potentially devastating impact on his patient to a basically positive and helpful one. Cousins reports that six months later, two thirds of the patient's tumors had disappeared.

Notice Cousins' emphasis on the partnership between the doctor and patient. Again, this relates back to shamanistic healing, in which the expectations invested in that relationship were often virtually the only ingredient in successful healings. Hopefully, such positive human dynamics will once again come to be included in the modern healer's legitimate range of therapeutic options.*

But I propose we go beyond the use of placebos (which in

---

* A study in the *Journal of Psychosomatic Research* reports that "... the personality of the therapist is crucial. The spiritually convinced, charismastic healer has all the qualities of a meditator, and physiological measurement demonstrates that such a healer induced the state of meditation in his patients."[10]

effect "trick" the patient into healing him or herself) to the direct exploration of the underlying powers which the placebo so dramatically taps.* The unexpected success rates of such modalities as autogenic training, biofeedback, visualization, hypnosis, meditation, and dream therapy, clearly demonstrate the immediate accessibility of one's own self-healing capacities. Beyond placebo, they point the way to a remarkable possibility: auto-placebo. Self-Actuated Healing.

If this new approach to personal health, the science/art of conscious self-healing, becomes prevalent in our society (and the burgeoning self-care movement seems to be a valid precursor), it will signal a fundamental change in the way health care is defined and accessed: *In the information age, self discovery is therapeutic, and knowledge is medicine.* Hospitals of the future will maintain healing libraries, and a variety of special spaces conducive to intensive personal growth therapies: crying rooms, chapels and meditation rooms, sensory deprivation tanks, conjugal sex accommodations, color environments, herb gardens, etc.

The reasons why such a change in our approach to health should be supported and promoted are numerous and compelling. They include economic and social, as well as personal benefits. Eight hundred dollars of the price of a new car goes to medical insurance for the company's workers![11] Along with the sheer cost of high-tech, allopathic medical intervention, the disturbing phenomenon of doctor-, drug-, and hospital-caused illness (termed "iatrogenesis") has now reached unacceptable levels, and has seriously eroded the public's confidence in the established health-care delivery system.[12]

After two centuries of monopoly by the Euro-American, patriarchal, allopathic medical establishment, and its at times ruthless suppression of alternative methods, the popular de-mystification of medical knowledge and democratization of its authority is now well underway, spurred on by self-help

---

* Placebo: (Latin) "I please"

groups, feminist health centers, self-care publications, electronic networking, and the relatively cooperative, supportive, and patient-empowering holistic health movement. The answer to the pending bankruptcy of Medicare may very well be Selfcare.

WHAT IS HEALTH?

Most people give little thought to the question of health until their symptoms and suffering inform them that it has been lost. Usually, "health" is understood to be merely the absence of discomfort and illness. When ailments do manifest, the common response is to place the body (and all too often the mind) under the control of a paid professional medical mechanic (a functionary of what Ken Pelletier calls the "pathology management industry"), and hope that he does the right thing, although his intervention options are sorely limited, primarily to chemicals and surgery. Both parties participate in an unquestioned, implicit arrangement which assumes complete passivity and subservience on the part of the patient.*

But perpetuating such a passive/negative relationship in the important issue of our own health does us a great disservice, and stifles our potential for realizing the wonderful, very real possibility of true optimum wellness. Real health is our natural birthright, and includes a tangible sense of wholeness, energy, joy, creativity, power, resilience, confidence, and a high level of performance of all our faculties and functions. The holistic philosophy contends that most people can experience this positive wellness, if they become knowledgeable about the strategies necessary to achieve and maintain it, and activated in practicing them. The pursuit of health becomes a long-term, dynamic process built into one's lifestyle, rather than an inconvenience based on the passive acceptance of whatever fate, or doctors dictate.

---

* A recent study showed that psychological and psychiatric language has five times as many terms implying "passivity" and "being acted upon" as it has terms implying "action," "self-organization" and "self-steering behavior."[13]

We also need to de-objectify health. Our materialistic society, with its expectation of instant results, has come to see health as just another consumer commodity, available through the "health care delivery system" for the right price. This commercialization of health has made us believe that health is a product, when in fact it is actually a personal, participatory experience. It's unfortunate that the notion of Self-Healing has become an almost alien concept in our society. This book, and others like it, aim to promote the realization of health as a way of being, a positive behavioral relationship to one's body, life and universe.

There is also a need for more encouraging and inspirational literature for the layperson on successful recovery from serious illness. It seems that anecdotal material is particularly effective in these cases, and it is offered here as both a contribution to an as-yet small body of literature, and an effort to help lift the prejudice, still prevalent within mainstream medicine, against such subjective, case-specific accounts.

WHAT IS HEALING?

Medicine consists of amusing the patient while nature cures the disease.   —*Voltaire*

REGENERATION. At the cellular level, healing entails the division, growth, and multiplication of individual cells, rebuilding or replenishing themselves in an orderly configuration which duplicates their ideal genetic design. This cellular renewal is a routine part of biological life: Virtually all the cells in your body will die and be replaced by others in the normal course of events. For blood cells the turnover time is less than two weeks, effectively amounting to a natural transfusion twice per month. Other types of body cells last longer, but it is a fact that, speaking from a purely physical point of view, you are not the same person you were just a few months or years ago. Knowing this is a good reason to be optimistic about self-healing. Rapid and complete regeneration is an everyday

---

* Healing in Old English is "Haelen"—to make whole.

process which you have been accomplishing all your life.

But since this cellular turnover involves the replacement of bodily mass, it should be obvious that the quality of the newly-assimilated building material is critical to the results. In other words, notwithstanding the institutionalized ignorance of these factors in "modern" medicine, *diet and nutrition are significant, primary variables in healing at the cellular level.* It seems a most curious inconsistency that the reductionist, material-based bio-medical sciences have failed to make the simple maxim, "you are what you eat" one of their guiding principles.

Simply to *eat* is to participate in one's own repair, although for the most part doctors tragically compromise that involvement by failing to educate patients about the importance of diet in healing, and in the case of hospitalization, by co-opting the patient's ability to determine quality, quantity and timing of meals. The results are often disastrous: People who should be marshaling one of the most important guides to health-recovery—their appetite—are attempting to "get well" on nutritionless and health-insulting, adulterated, manufactured food "products," selected primarily for their low cost, long shelf-life, cosmetic appearance, and ease of preparation, and served on a clockwork schedule that completely ignores organic individuality. This abominable situation is an insult to the intelligence and integrity of anyone seeking quality "health-care," and constitutes one of the more deplorable failures of the system. My suggestions for a simple and sane approach to a healthy diet follow in the chapter, "Eating To Heal."

The other side of cell regeneration is waste removal. The elimination of dead cells and the by-products of metabolism from the body is essential to good health. During times of healing, there are many ways in which we can act to maximize this internal cleansing process by supporting the optimal functioning of the organs of elimination (kidneys, lungs, colon, lymph system, and skin). Briefly, these methods include: the dietetic approach, in which certain foods and herbs known to be purifying are taken; fasting; aerobic exercise, which accelerates waste elimination (through sweating); skin brushing, and other forms of physical stimulation such as massage, and inversions. Colonic irrigation (enemas) can also be highly effective for internal cleansing.

The cellular view of life highlights another important variable that needs to be taken into account in questions of healing: Note that the difference between healthy cell regeneration and uncontrolled, (cancerous) cell profusion is that in the latter case, the *informing pattern of order* has not been successfully impressed on the wild cells. It is a premise of this book that although the non-physical source of this order may not yet, or ever, be identified by science, it can be *mediated by consciousness.* In other words, you are not only what you *eat,* but what you *think, believe,* and *feel,* as well.[14] Inasmuch as we can learn about the "mind-side" of the self-repair equation, we can make medicines of our thoughts, emotions, and visions, and true self-induced healing becomes not only a possibility, but in many cases, the "treatment" of choice.

Health is the consummation of a love affair of the organs of the body.   *—Plato*

SYSTEMIC BALANCE. One effect of the orderly, cooperative growth of numerous cells is the observable mending of tissue, organs and bones. But proper functioning at this level also entails a healthy relationship among the various systems which they comprise. For example, think of the complex interdependence of the circulatory and respiratory, the digestive and eliminative, and the nervous, endocrine, and immune systems. The maintenance or restoration of a dynamic, multi-dimensional, mutually informative equilibrium of systems (homeostasis) is crucial to any attempt at health improvement. (Norman Cousins calls this inter-system neuro-electro-chemical feedback process, "self-regulatory normalization.") Again, this is for the most part an automatic process, but this systemic interaction is also affected by mind and emotions. Therefore, balanced internal organic self-regulation is an enormous asset when healing is required. For example, people with Raynaud's disease could easily be taught to self-induce greater blood circulation to the extremities with muscle relaxation, breathing, and visualization techniques.

Note that whether we view healing from the cellular or systemic levels, both are *automatic,* and therefore ultimately nothing but *self*-healing. There is nothing inherent in any drug, surgical procedure, or other applied intervention that in itself accounts for cell growth, tissue repair, or restored organ function (although they may accelerate the desired results, mostly by creating metabolic circumstances favorable to the body's own repair mechanisms). The finest surgeon in the world knows that he can do no more than draw the edges of a wound together and hope that the body re-grows the living tissue to connect them. *Only the organism can repair the organism.* In other words, *all healing is self-healing.* The wise physician will always bear this in mind, and make every effort to support and encourage the innate healing powers of the patient, without which, his or her efforts are bound to be in vain.

RE-ENERGIZING. In eastern systems of healing, particularly the Chinese meridian/five-element theory, and the Indian Ayurvedic school, homeostasis and the important dynamic relationship among the many organ systems is understood to be essentially a question of energy flow. This is an entire dimension of our being that physical medicine has until now overlooked. Science has just begun to investigate the human energy field through Therapeutic Touch, Kirlian photography, brain wave research, nuclear-magnetic resonance (NMR), and the application of nuclear quantum-mechanical theories to neuro-biology.

There are numerous names for the "energy of life": Prana, Shakti, Kundelini, Chi, Orgone, Bio-magnetism, Plasma, Ether, etc. What is more important than what we call it, is the fact that for the first time in history, the general population has at its disposal the knowledge necessary to make deliberate and effective use of these inner resources. These practices have been known in their various indigenous cultures as Yoga, Pranayama, Tu Mo, Tantra, T'ai Chi Chuan, Kung Fu, Reiki, Aikido, Kum Nye, etc. Today in the West we have some early equivalent pscho-technologies, minus the religious overtones: Jacobsenian Progressive Muscle Relaxation, Isometrics, Therapeutic Touch, Polarity, Autogenic Training, Biofeedback, "Rebirthing," Visualization techniques, Sensory Deprivation, Hypnosis—all effective energy-generation or circulation techniques; all sciences, in the strict sense, with predictable results, experientially verifiable, if not yet quantifiable.

From Pythagoras, Hippocrates learned that health, as wholeness, means that the body and the soul must be examined together, that there are spiritual laws which human beings can ignore but only at their own peril, that human will ensures and completes the harmony between body, mind and soul, that complete human beings are those who have grasped the sense of this harmony and implemented it in their own lives, and this harmony means thinking correctly, and living correctly—according to the law. The ancient people appreciated the value of philosophy for their own life. For Pythagoras, harmony was the key term. Harmony holds it all or nothing is held. —Henry Skolimowski[15]

WHOLENESS. These then are the aspects of a working definition of *Conscious Self-Actuated Healing:*
- A dynamic quest for wholeness. The wise application of health-promoting strategies and lifestyle habits, including healthful diet, exercise, relaxation, cultivation of positive mental/emotional states, and spiritual receptivity.
- Intentional activation of, and cooperation with, one's innate natural body-repair mechanisms. The process of discovering what the system needs, providing it, and augmenting it with strong desire, positive expectation

and skillful imagery.

● Deliberate mobilization of biologic and subtle energies for optimizing one's natural recuperative powers. Effective use of intuition, will, and visionary capabilities to support healing.

HEALING IN CONTEXT: TRANSPERSONAL FACTORS. While this is a study of self-healing, it does not assume that human beings are islands of autonomy and self-sufficiency. Health cannot be maintained in an unhealthy environment, ecological or psychological; and there is no substitute for human touch, now being acknowledged by medical science as a legitimate healing intervention.[16]. (Even pets are important, as many special education, geriatric, and mental health workers are now re-discovering.) The focus of this work is on the inherent self-healing powers of the individual, but this is not meant to exclude any possible external positive influences, private or professional. It is always hoped that those seeking health will find strength and guidance from all potentially helpful sources, within and without.

The shamen of old knew that the whole family is the patient and the whole tribe is the healer. Today, in the age of the one-generation nuclear family, the contemporary special interest "support group" often effectively fills the vital function of a counsel of empathetic peers. The holistic therapist or counselor investigates the interpersonal context of health problems, and involves family, friends, and if necessary, co-workers, towards desired health-goals. Significant others are engaged for spiritual as well as logistical support, and the potential power of the collective belief system is enlisted. Good communication is healthy, and surely love is the closest thing we have to a universal medicine.

II.

AUTONOMOUS APPROACHES TO STRESS

Much has been written and said about stress in recent years, as the health implications of late twentieth century lifestyles become more evident. Thanks to the work of such pioneers as Dr. Hans Selye, Dr. Herbert Benson, Drs. Friedman and Rosenman, and Holmes and Rahe, stress is now recognized as a major factor in many disease states, and stress management and relaxation therapies, classes, and books are proliferating. This is a welcome development. We have adapted so readily to stressful habits that within a couple of generations, we've lost the memory and experience of a more natural and balanced existence. Today, real relaxation is one of the most universally needed and beneficial gifts we could give ourselves.

Stress was first clinically defined by Dr. Selye, who received the Nobel Prize in medicine for his ground-breaking work in this relatively new field. Selye, who cured himself of cancer, took a uniquely whole-systems approach to behavior and health. He reasoned that if we are to know how to get well, we need to understand the entire human process of "getting sick" itself, as opposed to analyzing only specific diseases and isolated symptoms. All stress-related disease, said Selye, is part of one's General Adaptation Syndrome, regardless of specific causes or effects. He was studying the body's inherent defense mechanisms, as opposed to its external enemies.

Selye defined stress as the full constellation of physiological responses of the organism to change. All of us have built-in self-regulatory mechanisms, mediated by the autonomic nervous system, that allow us to healthfully absorb or deflect some amount of challenge to our systems, physical or emotional. These include the universal body reactions of increased heart and breath rate, blood pressure, skin response, and various adjustments in the glandular and circulatory systems that optimize the efficiency of the muscles and other organs most immediately essential to self-protection and survival during such response. Even pain-deadening chemical triggers are released in the brain in preparation for a critical confrontation of one kind or another. The totality of these body reactions is one's stress level.

All these reactions are nature's original survival tools, equipping us to deal effectively with real-time challenges, as they have been occurring to human beings throughout the millennia of our evolution: dangerous predators, extreme weather changes, the fight for food, etc. At such times the self-preservation instincts of the primitive nervous system prepared the organism metabolically for one of two elementary responses: fight or flight.[1] When the appropriate response is taken, the stress reactions in the body are utilized positively, and one's adaptation to the stressor is successfuly completed.

In such instances stress can be seen as a positive and helpful force (called *eustress* by Selye), important to the creation of self-protective strategies and the maintenance of physical fitness. In sports, it is the *eustress* of competition that creates the metabolic potential which enables an athlete to excell. In fact, without a sufficient quota of this healthy brand of stress, we would all be weak invalids.

We can see then, that (notwithstanding the popular negative connotation assigned to the term) not all stress is "bad." It is when stress is unabated, and our response is inappropriate and/or unsuccessful in either removing the source, or ourselves from it, that stress itself becomes the debilitating factor (distress).

Unfortunately, modern civilized life presents all too many such no-win situations. A classic example is the harried office employee who incurs the wrath of her boss and has no real avenue of retaliation. Although the well-functioning, primitive nervous system responds to the confrontation with an infusion of adrenalin, various gastric secretions, increased muscle tone, skin moisture, heartbeat, etc., the modern circumstance allows no effective outlet for the resulting state of tension (i.e., most cannot *fight* their superiors, or *flee* their jobs.)* Domestic tensions, driving in traffic, financial pressures, and even watching the evening news can have the same effect: a perpetual state of preparedness, with no way out and no physical resolution of the over-stimulation.

Regardless of the cause, our bodies cannot indefinitely sustain a state of emergency preparedness. Breakdown occurs. If stressful conditions are not relieved, more serious disease, and eventually premature death can ensue. It has been estimated that up to eighty percent of all common illnesses have recognizable stress-related causes or contributing factors. Early symptoms of the General Adaptation Syndrome may include insomnia, anxiety, appetite loss or compulsive eating, headaches, muscle tension, digestive disorders, hypertension, glandular exhaustion, and similar complaints. A recent study reported in *Science* proved that cancer can be induced through stress in animals.[3]

The psychological costs of the inability to relax are also considerable: Unabated stress can jeopardize relationships and upset whole families. Frustration becomes cynicism, and over-aggressive behavior can foreshadow "Regressive Disequilibrium," including personality breakdown, and even suicide.[4]

* Researchers at SRI International have concluded that personality/job "mismatch" can be a significant source of stress and chronic illness. Look for greater corporate investments in stress reduction for employees and management in the nineties, as the real costs of business stress—in medical expenses, productivity, and employee moral—become acknowledged.

Ingrained neuroses and irrational beliefs about oneself can be a source of stress. Inferiority complexes and performance anxiety can become hidden, life-long stressors and may require skillful cognitive intervention to overcome. At best, life in a state of chronic stress becomes a constant battle against disease and despair.

Possible reactions to excess stress are determined by person-specific variables and predisposing factors such as heredity, medical history, lifestyle, cultural conditioning, and psychological type. The meaning and impact, and even the value of stress in one's life, depend upon the effectiveness (or lack) of personal coping strategies, be they automatic or practiced, native or acquired. It is significant that one man's stress can be another man's eustress. Some people are at risk for chronic stress burnout (ironically, medical doctors rate high on the list), while others enjoy stress immunity, a natural hardiness to the vicissitudes of life.[5] Most people can be taught coping skills, but it's a unique process for each individual. No two persons stress-reduction requirements, strategies, or responses are necessarily the same.

No doctor can "cure" you of stress. Stress management is virtually synonymous with self-care. When the nature of chronic over-stress and its effects on personal well-being are understood, stress management proves to be the quintessential self-healing project. The holistic approach is characteristically multi-dimensional, as are the origins of stress-related problems.

HOLISTIC STRESS REDUCTION

... anxiety and relaxation are mutually exclusive. That is, anxiety does not, cannot exist when the muscles are truly relaxed.

—*Barbara Brown*, Stress & The Art of Biofeedback

The opposite of the stress response has been termed the Relaxation Response (RR) by Dr. Herbert Benson.[6] It amounts to a direct reversal of the physiological stress indicators mentioned above, the elimination of many stress-induced symptoms, and frequently, a corresponding sense of relief.

The best news about the Relaxation Response is that it can be self-induced. A practical example would be the over-stressed waitress using progresive muscle relaxation on her break to abate (or better yet, avoid) an on-the-job tension headache.

All of the anti-stress strategies described below aim for the voluntary self-induction of the RR at will, as well as long-term stress-hardiness. Their successful application depends upon correct training and regular use. Often, a combination of approaches greatly enhances their effectiveness, as with biofeedback and autogenic techniques.

Note: An effective relaxation program will reduce the need for various stress-control drugs, sedatives, and pain medications. Because this can turn a normal dosage into an over-dose, people on medications should only pursue these methods under regular medical supervision.

PROGRESSIVE MUSCLE RELAXATION

One of the most reliable and popular stress reduction techniques, Progressive Muscle Relaxation (PMR) was first developed in the late 1920's by Edmund Jacobson, M.D. It's a simple physically-based exercise/relaxation cycle which capitalizes on the two-way relationship between mind an muscles. The method is best learned by hearing the instructions while practicing as with a tape recording or skilled narrator. After the technique is memorized, audible instructions are no longer necessary.

The Jacobsonian method starts with a paradoxical approach: Muscle tension is deliberately increased first. This powerful flexing highlights the sensations of tension and helps develop awareness and control over isolated local muscle groups. It also expends excess adrenalin in the system, and uses up residual nervous energy.

This "isometric" flexing can be done in increasing degrees of intensity, enabling one to explore and expand one's possible strength potentials. Strong contraction of the muscles also expells metabolic waste products from the cells, and stimulates and tonifies blood vessels. (People with cardio-vascular and circulatory disease, glaucoma, migraines, and other pressure-sensitive conditions should do flexing exercises only moderately.)

The relaxation phase follows immediately after the tightening of the muscles in question. Opening the muscle cells allows an influx of fresh oxygen and nutrients. Muscle areas are worked separately and in progression (usually from the top down). Isolation of muscle groups is enhanced. This provides a clear feeling of the great difference one can make in releasing specific areas of muscle tension. The student is encouraged to sense this difference and to continue "letting go" to deeper levels of relaxation. The contrast created by going through the full range of possible muscle activity, tense to relaxed, makes this method immediately satisfying and self-validating. In this way, one learns to *recognize tension,* and *choose relaxation.*

Following this pattern throughout the body, all the muscles are systematically contracted and released, and all tension is replaced with deep relaxation. The attention is placed on the resulting sensations of softness, warmth, openness, etc. Jacobson observed (and you will too, if you try it!) that mental anxiety or agitation is virtually incompatible with this deep muscular relaxation. The more the technique is practiced, the more accessible, quick, and profound the effects, both physical and mental.

AUTOGENIC TRAINING

As a man thinketh in his heart, so he is.   —*Proverbs 23:7*

Autogenic training ("A.T.," or simply "autogenics") has similarities to progressive muscle relaxation. Entire limbs are relaxed at once, and sub-vocal training phrases are added, consisting of first person, present tense, affirmative descriptions of the bodily sensations of relaxing. For example: "My right arm feels heavy and warm." All body parts should be experienced in this way. Other autogenic induction phrases include: "My heartbeat feels slow and calm" and "My breathing feels soft and light." These formulas directly access the autonomic nervous system, and create a self-induced Relaxation Response with measurable results in all the typical body indicators. Imagery and relaxing music can also be used to reinforce the effect. "A.T." is an excellent biofeedback training method, and works synergistically with that modality.

As a healthful self-therapy, autogenic training is particularly applicable to disorders of the respiratory and gastro-intestinal tracts, and the cardio-vasular and endocrine systems. Excellent results have also been obtained in cases of insomnia, anxiety, phobias, headache, bronchial asthma, chronic constipation, and a variety of neuro-motor disfunctions, including epilepsy, stuttering, torticollis, bruxism, etc.[7] It also works well in conjunction with cognitive methods, such as systematic desensitization.

BREATHING TECHNIQUES

Give me your tired, your poor, your huddled mases yearning to breath free. — *The Statue of Liberty*

Breathing is a unique function in the organism, owing to its property of being a primary life-sustaining, involuntary reflex which is also readily subject to voluntary control. This dual nature of the breath makes it a perfect faculty for use in the investigation of the mind/body interface, and places it squarely in the center of the self-regulation sciences.

Notions of the fundamental and all-pervasive importance of the breath have been built into our language: The medical prefix *pneumo*, pertaining to the lungs, originally comes from the Greek word for soul or spirit. To take in this spirit is "in-spiring." In Genesis, God imparted life to Adam by *breathing* into him. To *expire*, is to die. And the word *con-spiracy* derives from "breathing together."

We all know from experience that fear, anxiety, and emotional turmoil render one's breathing tight, shallow and rapid. Not everyone realizes, however, that deliberate, slow, deep breathing, or even simply placing the awareness on the breath, can reverse these negative mental states. This approach has also been successfully applied in self-controlling high blood pressure,[8] and chronic pain.[9]

From a strictly physiological perspective, the importance of healthy breathing cannot be over-emphasized, for the breath functions to supply all the cells in the body with oxygen (and hence, energy), as well as removing the toxic by-products of metabolism, particularly carbon dioxide.

Poor breathing habits can be linked to lung diseases, digestive and circulatory disorders, and a variety of oxygen-deprivation complaints, including headaches, cold extremities, weak muscles, chronic fatigue, and many metabolic deficiencies and auto-toxic conditions.[11] There is good evidence supporting the theory that certain types of malignancies are at least in part related to an under-supply of oxygen on a cellular level. Breathing also represents our only means of assimilation of negative ions, which seem to be important to many aspects of health.[10]

Many doctors seem unaware that numerous disorders can often be alleviated by correcting the patient's posture, relaxing the diaphragm, strengthening the abdomen, and cleaning and expanding the capacity of the lungs with proper breathing exercises. But there are other dimensions of breath awareness and breath control techniques that go well beyond the muscular and structural benefits of conventional respiratory therapy. In deep relaxation techniques, close attention to breathing patterns elicits psycho-physiological effects that can be greatly healing, not the least of which is relaxation far surpassing anything possible through muscular approaches alone.

The function of breathing is intimately related to our psycho-emotional life, creating a "breath language" that to the astute observer is every bit as revealing as our body language: We sigh with relief, gasp in astonishment, hold the breath with fear, choke with sadness, and explode in anger. Variations in breathing depth and rhythm closely parallel our thoughts and feelings, and directly relate to all other metabolic systems.[12] And the latest research on brain hemisphere dominance tends to confirm the yogic theory that the alternation of the flow of breath between the left and right sides of the breathing passages is another important indicator of operant modes of perception and behavior.[13]

Proper breathing and breath control are emphasized in virtually all meditation traditions. In yoga, the breath is said to be the key to health and long life, due to its relationship to the intake and circulation of "prana," the universal energy of life ("first unit"= *pra;* "energy"= *na*). In oriental medicine, coordination and control of the breath energy (Japanese: *ki,* Chinese: *chi)* is seen as essential to health, and the martial arts use it in the generation of power and stamina.

BREATHING EXERCISES

The next few pages contain detailed instructions on various breath techniques which I have learned from many yoga, meditation and healing teachers, and practiced over the last twenty years. They are also available and explained in greater detail in several good books, included in the source list at the back of this one.

These techniques require some study and practice before benefits become significant. Some amount of preparation is necessary. In the exercises and breathing techniques that follow, several premises are assumed:

● You should be empty. Don't do deep breathing exercises within two or three hours of eating. Empty the bladder and bowels as well.

● Clothing should be loose-fitting and comfortable.

● As with all relaxation and meditation practices, the surroundings should be quiet and free of distractions. Breathing exercises are best done outdoors, or by an open window (if you are in a non-polluted environment).

● People with high blood pressure, heart diseases, or disorders of the central nervous system should refrain from rigorous or deep breathing exercises, or consult with their doctor about the appropriateness of these methods to their condition.

● The best way to learn these techniques is to hear them while practicing, so pre-recording these instructions is recommended.

If you are new to breathing exercises, do not be fooled by their simplicity. Practice daily, even for just a few weeks, and you will be surprised to discover how healing these techniques can be.

DIAPHRAGMATIC BREATHING. Also known as the "complete breath," this procedure gives a fuller awareness and use of the various anatomical structures involved in proper breathing. Most people breathe far too shallowly and with only a small portion of their lungs, specifically the upper half or third. This is due to a variety of reasons: over-eating, poor posture, tight clothing, chronic tension, and self-consciousness concerning weight, particularly in women. For men, improper breathing also comes from the military model: stomach in, chest out, chin in. This too contradicts our natural breathing mechanisms and creates negative effects on health.

The area of the lungs most adversely affected by common poor breathing habits is the lower lobes. Due to the lack of movement and fresh air in this region, it is the location most susceptible to infection (pneumonia), fluid build-up, tissue atrophy, etc. Complete diaphragmatic breathing involves becoming aware of, and using the lower lobes first. This is done by exercisng the muscles of the diaphragm and abdomen, maximizing their involvement in deep breathing.

A good position to learn complete diaphragmatic breathing is supine, with the knees bent. Loosen all constricting clothing at the waistline. Place your hand over the navel. Begin by simply noticing how the abdomen rises and falls naturally in this position as you breathe normally. Confirm for yourself that when you inhale, the belly swells and expands, lifting your hand up. The deeper the inbreath, the greater the outward displacement of the abdomen. As natural as this movement is, it may come as something of a revelation if you have been used to thinking of "taking a deep breath" as synonymous with sucking the stomach in. If you are laying on your back and relaxed, quite the opposite will occur.

Begin to exaggerate this distension of the belly with each breath, making the inhalations deeper. Your abdomen is like a balloon being pumped up. Anatomically, the diaphragm muscle is pushing the belly up and out of the way, and pulling the bottom of the lungs, stretching them longer, down the length of the body. When you are full, hold for a moment, and then let the exhalation suddenly rush out of you. Practice belly breathing for a few minutes. Get a feeling for breathing from and into the belly. This is the first of three distinct movements involved in the Complete Breath.

The second movement is added after the abdominal inhalation is complete. It involves taking air into the thoracic cavity proper, by expanding the rib cage. You should practice these two steps in sequence: First inhale abdominally, then continue to take in more air by expanding the chest. Once again, exhalation is accomplished automatically by simply relaxing and letting the breath fall out.

The third component of the Complete Breath is the lifting of the upper costal structure (collar bones and shoulders), and the filling of the top-most regions of the respiratory tract. Put the head back and pull the air into the sinus cavities. You should have the feeling that you have maximized your vital capacity by both stretching the lungs lengthwise and expanding them outward, sequentially, in all three sections described. Again, allow the outbreath to follow freely. This completes the diaphragmatic breathing cycle. It can be highly therapeutic when practiced repeatedly, several times daily, either exclusively, or as preparation for other self-care routines, such as yoga, meditation, autogenics, etc. Positive benefits should be noticeable within a couple of weeks, if not immediately.

THE CLEANSING BREATH. This procedure purges the lungs of stale waste gases and makes the alveoli (minute air sacks) more pliant. It also has the secondary benefits of stimulating the heart and digestive organs.

Thoroughly and somewhat forcefully expel all the air from the lungs through the mouth by compressing first the abdomen, then the chest and shoulders, so that all your air is pushed out. This strongly curves the body forward. You should feel like you are squeezing out the last bit of exhaled air from the bottom up. It helps to think of the contraction beginning at the genital muscles and progressively tightening upward, as when emptying a tube of toothpaste. This is the purification phase. (If it makes you cough, it means you need it, for irritating particulate deposits are being loosened into the bronchial passages. Moderate the exercise according to your tolerance, but plan on practicing regularly until the lungs are cleared and the cough reaction ceases. See your doctor if it doesn't.)

Then relax and let the air rush in through the nostrils. As with the Complete Breath above, continue the inhalation by deliberately distending the belly, then expanding the rib cage and finally lifting the upper chest and shoulder area. Take in as much air as possible by both lengthening and expanding the entire respiratory cavity. Then exhale and relax. This is the revitalizing phase.

After following this cycle a few times, hold the inbreath while thoroughly relaxing all the muscles in the body (Progressive Muscle Release). This infuses a great amount of oxygen directly into the brain and central nervous system (it not being needed by the body muscles at rest). After about fifteen seconds of holding the breath (while relaxing the body, particularly the neck, shoulders, and abdomen), let the air rush out and allow the breath to move freely and normalize as you observe the effects.

If you find the results of this deep cleansing breath beneficial, use it regularly. Your lung capacity and retention time will gradually increase. If you feel mild adverse effects, such as nausea or dizziness, modify the depth of the inhalation, and reduce the time of the held breath. Mental "centering" techniques will also help (see section on

Meditation). Within a few weeks, you should be able to build up your tolerance and capacity for deep breathing, and notice positive results, such as a feeling of lightness, greater mental clarity, more energy, less sleep requirements, and relief from minor or even major respiratory-related symptoms, as mentioned previously. The cleansing breath routine also tends to keep the digestive system in good shape, especially when done in conjunction with inversion practices, such as shoulder stands, or the use of a slant board.

PASSIVE BREATH AWARENESS. Passive Breath Awareness (PBA) is the opposite and complimentary breathing practice to the active breath control techniques described above. In this case, no effort of will is imposed upon the natural, automatic rhythm of the breath. Instead the idea is to keep the attention focused as closely and consistently as possible on the intake and outflow of the breath *without influencing it.* Whereas in the active exercises, we decide when to push or pull the breath through its cycles, in PBA, we observe what the breath wants to do by itself, and when, as it seeks and settles into its own internally measured pace. It's a way of consciously connecting with one of our deeper sources of biological rhythm within. The feeling is one of complete, attentive surrender to your own metabolism.

There are definite, predictable physiological effects of this "effortless effort": By getting out of the way of the breath (but staying closely aware of it), it automatically slows down. So do the pulse rate and other bodily functions.[14] It's a paradoxical approach to accessing the autonomic nervous system, amounting to control by letting go of control. Here's how it's done:

The focus for the mind to fix upon in PBA can be one of several discernable physiological sensations associated with breathing, such as the rising and falling of the abdomen, or the feeling of the air passing by the tips of the nostrils. You may also try developing an internal sense of the movement of the diaphragm muscle itself, as this is the actual physiological location of the origin of the breath. (You'll learn more about this center in later sections on core relaxation and chakra meditation.)

Choosing a breath focal point, observe it very carefully, but as a *passive witness:* intensely interested in the feeling of breathing, but not interfering with it in any way. Instead, *let the air breathe you.* Keeping your attention only at the chosen focus, explore in the light of one-pointed concentration, the timing, duration, and sensations of breathing, while allowing it to become more deeply automatic with each cycle. Sense how closely you can attend to the subtle changes of each breath as it comes, being taken by it like a surfer on a wave, without resistance, hesitation, anticipation, or clinging.

A key part of the practice is to follow the outbreath as long and as far as it will take you, by continually relaxing into it. By going with the breath, you will be pleasantly surprised to discover how deep the experience can become.

The difficultly in this practice lies in learning how to mentally stay with it long enough to create and notice the results. Since the habitual thinking mind is not used to remaining trained on a single object for any length of time, particularly something as seemingly uninteresting as the breath, it usually quickly wanders away to other places, times, and images. All meditative and internal self-regulation techniques require that this restlessness of mind be gradually replaced by a voluntary, clear, simple concentration of awareness on one object for a chosen length of time.

For this reason, useful concentration methods have been developed to free the mind from distractions, and help keep consciousness and breath together. The most common of these involves simply counting the breaths: Mentally assign successive numbers, from one to ten, to each in-and-out breath cycle. You may very well discover that your "train of thought" persists in derailing before reaching your destination (the number ten !). When it does, simply start over. When you can reach ten, try counting backwards down to one. Repeat this routine many times until you can keep your mind focused solely on the breath, at will, for ten minutes or longer. It may help to actually visualize the numbers written in the air before you (eyes closed). In this way, you will gradually develop and sustain the necessary concentration to practice breath awareness and other healing, deep consciousness techniques.

Other focusing devices for breathing include "labeling" the components of the breath with words, traditionally, but not necessarily with spiritual connotations; or, as in the Theravadan Buddhist tradition, by mentally noticing *("knowing")* the length, quality and other distinguishing characteristics of each breath in turn.

The final and most profound phase of PBA involves the investigation of the distinct momentary pause between breaths, when breathing actually stands still. This occurs at the "bottom" of the exhalation, before it turns into an inhalation. We call this the "Stillpoint," and it constitutes a potential for experiencing complete non-agitation, or "absorbtion." The value of consciously investigating this ephemeral internal event cannot be over-emphasized, for it leads to alterations of brain and body states that are intrinsically healing and growth promoting. The way to induce these states is to "enter" the Stillpoint.

When an exhalation is occurring, simultaneously relax all limbs and muscles as in the Progressive Muscle Release. When all the breath has fallen out of you, relax again, into a deeper level of body and breath passivity. Drop all residual tension on the finest level, and open to your own inner energy. Do this over and over again, each time you finish exhaling, but make no effort to either hasten or extend the Stillpoint with force or control. Simply wait for it to come, and then get completely absorbed in that moment of absolute stillness. No matter how fleeting it may be in clock time, the subjective experience of the Stillpoint can become vast and deep. Simply let it happen as it will. It helps to observe and *label* the Stillpoint as a third component, as you did the other two (inbreath & outbreath). Words like "Now," "One," or "Home," can be used to mark this moment of spacious inner tranquility.

You can also use imagery to "open up" the Stillpoint experience: During exhalation, imagine feeling like a feather gently settling down a deep well. At the moment of contact (the bottom of the out-breath), feel as if a trap door opens beneath you and you continue to float down to a lower level. This has the effect of effortlessly extending the Stillpoint experience, adding dimension each time it comes around, and making deeper inner states of awareness and peace more accessible with every practice session. This method is one of the ways in which yogis in India have learned to slow the heart, turn off pain, alter body temperature and accomplish other internal controls without the use of drugs.[15]

BIOFEEDBACK

Biofeedback training involves the use of sensitive electronic instruments that monitor subtle body changes and amplify them audibly or visually, enabling the subject to learn auto-regulation of metabolic functions that are usually below the threshold of conscious awareness. These include heart rate, blood pressure, skin temperature, brainwave activity, fine muscle tone, breath rate, etc. Given the state of the art today, virtually any detectable body activity can be amplified and input through the conscious mind/body feedback loop, rendering it subject to voluntary influence. Even the firing of single muscle or nerve cells can be detected, an ability which has made it apparent that humans can voluntarily affect the functions of the smallest discrete units of organic life within the body.

Although biofeedback is barely twenty years old, it has started a revolution in the health sciences, firmly establishing the importance of awareness, volition, interior concentration, subliminal perception, and other complex mental processes as significant variables in questions of internal controls, stress management, and health recovery. Disorders reported to respond to electromyogram (EMG) feedback alone include: Asthma, hypertension, bruxism, intestinal disorders (ulcers, colitis, spasms of muscles and sphincters), menstrual distress, pain, stroke, paralysis, hyperkinesis, dyskinesia, spasticity, cerebral palsy, spasmodic torticollis, migraine, anxiety, phobias, hyperactivity, insomnia, alcoholism, depression, and more.[16]

In understanding biofeedback, it is important to realize that the technological devices used are merely sophisticated electronic mirrors. They do nothing but relect our own remarkable organic sensitivity. The subtle metabolic changes we monitor through biofeedback are always taking place in response to our outer and inner environments. The instrument merely makes this fine level of auto-regulation more apparent to the conscious senses, and hence, more accessible to voluntary control. In fact, a main objective of biofeedback training is the elimination of the external amplification (the instrument) after self-regulation is functionally internalized. No other single modality so clearly illustrates the potentials of autonomous, self-induced healing. As pioneer researcher Barbara Brown puts it, "The patient is no longer the object of the treatment, he is the treatment!"

OTHER STRESS REDUCTION STRATEGIES

Differing, but quite compatible with the meditative approach, the cognitive methods of stress management depend upon the individual's ability to assess and deliberately change his or her mental patterns and behavior. These systematic psychological strategies include values clarification, goal setting, thought-stopping, communication skills, assertiveness training, time management, systematic desensitization and pain inoculation. The cognitive approach requires insight into one's habitual self-defeating psychological behaviors and the knowledge of how to alter them through training. Although such skills have been customarily developed through the traditional therapeutic relationship with counselors and psychologists, they are largely self-reliant techniques, and the material is now well presented in workbook form, such as the one by McKay, Davis, and Fanning (1981). Cognitive methods are very compatible with meditation and introspective modalities such as journal writing and dream therapy.

Another tactic among the holistic stress reduction options that has recently begun to gain attention is the use of humor and laughter. Now that Norman Cousins, Raymond Moody and Bernie Siegel have given voice to the notion, we can begin to enjoy ourselves in the name of health! No doubt there are neuro-chemical explanations for the effects of laughter on the nervous system. It certainly makes us breathe deeply and take in huge amounts of oxygen! I'm sure strong laughter induces bicameral brain functioning as well, as evidenced by the peak-like nature of the experience. It is also a tension-releasing physical/emotional catharsis that causes a general shutdown of our ego defenses. Next time you need an excuse to let yourself laugh, remember that it's better than pills and bills!

PHYSICAL APPROACHES. The primary focus of this investigation of stress reduction has been on non-physical factors, because their significance has been until now greatly underestimated. Let it not be assumed, however, that physical stress reduction activites are any less important: muscle tension can be directly relieved through stretching and self massage; the stress resiliency of the circulatory system benefits from a wide variety of cardio-vascular exercise, such as swimming, walking, running, bicycling, and racquet sports; and diet can be optimized to reduce stress (see section on food). Even sex can play an important role in this kind of self-healing. The holistic approach entails a constellation of autonomous activities that together act to bring all of one's being into harmony. Let the earnest seeker of health and peace choose intelligently among a range of inner as well as outer self-care methods. Positive results are bound to follow.

III.

EATING TO HEAL

No investigation of self-healing would be complete without a discussion of diet. Notwithstanding the conspicuous silence on the subject from the mainstream medical establishment, much has been written and said about the importance of diet to health, from a varity of sources. In some instances, not all the information is helpful:

● Some "experts" unholistically over-emphasize the importance of diet, as if it were the *only* determining factor in health, whereas exercise, stress management, relaxation, a healthy environment, and social and spiritual nurturance are equally important.

● Many prescribe one type of diet universally, failing to take into account individual differences in condition, heredity, geography, physiology, and lifestyle.

● Intelligent eating is far simpler than some systems would have us think. It's only because we have strayed so far from what nature intended for our food, that authoritarian, esoteric, and complicated "diets" are so frequently adopted in the place of sound thinking, careful observation, common sense, and personal intuition.

The following is not an attempt to document or detail the intimate relationship between diet, pathology, and healing. That has been accomplished quite well in books and periodicals, and continues to make news with growing frequency.

Rather, here is a summary of some fifteen years of study and experience in natural diet, and the distillation of a few basic and important principles of relevance to all, especially those wishing to maximize their own internal healing potentials.

NATURAL FOOD

What should we eat to get well? The same things we should eat to *stay* well, and live a long and disease-free life: organic grains, vegetables, fruit, beans, seeds, nuts, herbs, grasses, roots, and the juices thereof.

The human body is the product of billions of years of co-evolution with the environment. Only very recently have we radically altered our ancient ecological relationship to our own food source, to our great disadvantage and incalculable expense. It has taken a tragic kind of blindness for us to go so far astray so suddenly. In the two generations since the industrialization of food (in the forties and fifties), can be found large numbers of people who, in their whole lives, will rarely (if ever) enjoy the health-enhancing benefits of eating fresh, whole, unadulterated, unprocessed, *natural* food, for any meaningful amount of time. Indeed, given the low-nutritional, and high-synthetic content of most processed, preserved supermarket and fast-food fare, it is a testimonial to the miraculous survivability of the human organism that many people are alive today, in spite of what they eat. Many are in this predicament out of ignorance, some due to poverty. Most know better, but are simply enslaved by bad eating habits.

Suffering a loss of health, and *not* attempting to support your recovery with an optimum diet is like driving with the brakes on. Unfortunately this is still how most ill Americans behave: as if they really didn't want to get well. Rare are those who, after learning of the folly of their ways, are willing to acknowledge their transgressions of the ageless laws of nature and commit themselves to change. Those that can are frequently the ones who are most able to heal themselves.

By natural we mean close to the earth, in form, and in time. It is not natural to attempt to chemically extend the "shelf-life" of organic substances indefinitely. To do so and expect such inert products to sustain *real* life is sheer folly. The further a food is from its original state, the less healthy it is to eat. Natural means fresh, unsprayed, unwaxed, ungassed, and non-irradiated.

Home-grown sprouted seeds, legumes and grasses, and freshly-ground whole grain flours are the best examples of *live* natural foods: they still contain the nucleus of life, the living germ. The ultimate test for live food is: Will it grow when moistened and left alone? If so, we know that such foodstuffs contain the full complement of vitamins, enzymes, and vital energies necessary to generate and sustain organic life. These essential components are more or less sacrificed by processing, preserving, storing, and even cooking.

This is not to say that cooking or preserving food is unnatural or unnecessary! Obviously, certain very beneficial grains, beans and vegetables are completely indigestible uncooked. Equally necessary, especially in the temperate and cold climates, is the need to insure a reliable supply of food during the non-growing seasons. However, it is safe to say that most Americans do not eat enough raw vegetables and fruit (important sources of fiber, vitamins, and minerals) and often cook the nutrients out of their foods.

Cooking procedures have a significant impact on the quality of the food we ultimately ingest, and consequently on our health. In terms of their ability to preserve the perishable micro-nutrients so essential to health, and prevent the production of toxic by-products, the following methods are listed in descending order of preference: pressure cooking, steaming, baking, boiling, pan frying, charcoal grilling, and smoking. The last three tend to destroy vitamins most readily and produce carcinogenic carbonized by-products.[1]

Cooking utensils should be stainless steel, glass, cast iron, clay, or unchipped enamel. Avoid aluminum, which is a soft metal that easily reacts with hot food and contaminates it with aluminum oxide, a poison. It has recently been linked to Alzheimer's disease.[2] "Teflon" and other synthetic coatings also tend to migrate into food, and should not be used.

Freezing, home canning, and drying are the best methods of preserving natural food. The use of artificial preservatives, chemical anti-oxidants and inhibitors, or the practice of stripping the perishable components from the product is highly counter-productive in terms of nutrition. This rules out most packaged products found in the average store.

By organic we mean food that has grown in soil unpolluted by pesticides, chemical fertilizers, and other man-made contaminants. Such food is becoming increasingly more difficult to obtain commercially, making it all the more attractive to produce privately.

Even with the wide range of opinions on food and health, it is now generally agreed that certain substances definitely impair human health in anything but very modest quantities, and should be avoided or greatly controlled in the diet. Sugar, fat, cholesterol, salt, caffeine, and alcohol are among the most common offenders.[3]

Conversely, certain special foods are often recommended by natural health practitioners for their specific preventive and health-enhancing properties. Sprouts provide Vitamin C and chlorophyll, a liver cleanser and anti-cancer agent. Nutritional yeast is high in "B" vitamins, protein enzymes, and the important trace minerals chromium and selenium. Garlic is nature's strongest antibiotic and contact antiseptic. Sea kelp is an excellent source of iodine and trace minerals, and molasses has iron. Bee pollen is said to provide valuable enzymes. Cayenne pepper is a blood purifier and stimulant. Rose hips, parsley, and acerola berries are among the richest sources of Vitamin C. Lemon juice cleanses the liver, while cranberry juice helps purify the kidneys and bladder. Cultured, natural yogurt contains live enzymes that aid digestion. Soy lecithin reduces cholesterol and therefore helps prevent heart and circulatory problems. It also provides choline, needed to form vital neurotransmitters in the brain. In addition, hundreds of herbs have been used for centuries, throughout the world, for their specific curative effects on various common ailments. At least one highly respected and reputable contemporary herbalist, Dr. John Christopher, maintains that there is an herbal remedy for every illness known to man.[4]

It is noteworthy that for the most part, these natural, whole health aids and remedies are completely benign. There is little risk of over-dosage, dangerous combinations, or serious side-effects, as with "chemical equivalents," or distillations of "active ingredients." This is because nature always works in context, and material scientific analysis will never account for all the components of life. *Whole* food is more than just the sum of its parts, and usually better for us.

SUPPLEMENTS

As to the question of vitamin and mineral supplements— advocates of natural diet face a peculiar paradox: The expensive, high-tech, packaged powders, capsules and tablets commonly known as "vitamins," are the end-product of considerable processing, hardly resembling their original sources. How can their popularity among health and natural food proponents be reconciled with a dietary philosophy that claims to be close to nature and rely on whole foods? And are supplements really necessary if one is "eating right"?

Vitamin users reply that in an ideal, pristine environment, living a truly natural lifestyle, we would not need to supplement our diets. Unfortunately, just living in an industrialized society, in the contaminated environment of today, virtually guarantees deficiencies in our food and in our abilities to thoroughly absorb nutrients, and necessitates the use of concentrated food substances, grown and processed under rigorously controlled conditions (i.e. vitamins). Here's why:

SOIL DEPLETION & POLLUTION. Due to large-scale mono-crop cultivation, erosion, decades of accumulated chemical fertilizers and insecticides, and such man-made anomalies as acid rain, much of the soil from which our food comes is badly deficient and toxic. Such soil either lacks the full complement of nutrients for the produce to assimilate (such as the vital trace mineral selenium), or counteracts them with toxic anti-nutrient pollutants, such as DDT, which tends to destroy vitamins and stress the immune system.

HYBRID STRAINS. In an ideal world, the fruit and vegetables we find at the produce sections of our supermarkets would be cultivated for maximum nutritive value. But marketing motivations dictate that produce be bred for durability, uniformity, speed, color, and even for shape. The results are "products" that ship well, ripen slowly, and look sexy under fluorescent lighting, but which require ever-increasing doses of fertilizer to grow, are susceptible to disease, and are nutritionally defunct and tasteless.

HARVESTING PRACTICES. To compound the problem, in order to accommodate the rigors of long-distance distribution, produce is often harvested prematurely, by-passing the sun-ripening process, and sacrificing the very final-stage nutrients that nature prepares to sustain her own new-born seed. Some fruit, such as bananas, are force-ripened with gas after shipping. Thin skinned vegetables and fruit, such as cucumbers and apples, are often coated with paraffin, a non-digestible petro-chemical, to slow down deterioration and lend a more appealing look. Leafy vegetables such as lettuce are treated with sulfites to retard oxidation. (This adversely affects the human nervous system, particularly of asthmatics and other metabolically sensitive people.)

ADULTERATION. The next enemies of nutrition are the additives: colorings, preservatives, emulsifiers, texturizers, extenders, inhibitors, antioxidants, etc: all anti-nutrient non-food ingredients that strain our natural digestive powers, accumulate in the body, and deplete or counteract the body's vitamin quotas. Other known vitamin-antagonists include coffee, tobacco, chocolate, chlorinated water, and antibiotics. Many environmental pollutants, such as lead, DDT, sulfur-dioxide and the ever-present auto emission, carbon-monoxide, similarly impair nutrient assimilation or over-tax the normal supply. (CO gas inactivates the oxygen-carrying capacity of hemoglobin and creates an anemic condition.)

LOSSES IN COOKING: As mentioned, even when we succeed in securing pure, fresh, wholesome food, we can sabotage its potential benefits through unskillful preparation. The problem is even more serious at commercial eateries, where we all-too-often expect to find nourishment and sustenance in spite of such food-destroying practices as boiling vegetables, recycling frying oil, reheating with hot-lights and microwaves, and the "dipping" and spraying of salad vegetables. Only the few most hearty and abundant nutrients can survive such treatment intact.

FOOD COMBINING: The combinations in which foods are eaten can determine their nutritional availability and ultimate value to the body. This is because different types of foods call for different digestive secretions. The sugars in raw fruit, for instance, are processed by different enzymes than the carbohydrates and proteins of grains and vegetables. Taking them together confuses the digestive glands and dilutes their secretions, leading to incomplete breakdown, poor assimilation, putrefaction, and gaseous by-products. Even taking too much liquid during a meal dilutes the digestive juices. In these ways, good ingredients can combine to create bad effects. To prevent this, here are some general, healthy food-combining rules:

- Don't combine raw fruits and raw vegetables.
- Don't combine milk products and grains or beans.
- Don't combine proteins or leafy greens with acid fruits.[5]

Add to these problems the destructive effects of fast eating, over-eating, and eating under emotional stress, and the case is well made for the kind of nutritional insurance provided by vitamin and mineral supplements.

We see than that food quality, quantity, preparation, and combinations all have a bearing on the ultimate value and health-effects of what we eat. While diet is not the only variable, a clear and comprehensive view of the question reveals how vital it is to our prospects for healing. Let those who earnestly desire optimum health look to the dinner plate for an opportunity to improve themselves.

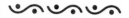

IV.

THERAPEUTIC FASTING

(Day 7)—It's been a week since I've had a bite to eat, but I haven't felt this good in years. My whole body feels clean and efficient, my mind calm and lucid. With so much new-found space inside where digesting bulk used to be, breathing has become a whole new experience. My sinuses feel like vast, spacious canyons swept by oceans of fresh air.

I'm sleeping less, but very deeply. Having beautiful, vivid dreams, and waking up feeling reborn. I'm 36 years old, and it seems like I've been getting younger every day. I wonder why the benefits of fasting have been so completely overlooked by our society...

Although nowadays the common response to sickness is usually to "take something," a growing number of people believe we could do well to try the alternative. Therapeutic fasting seems to be an excellent health restorative practice, for improving one's general condition, as well as for specific curative applications. Its value in self-healing far exceeds the current public and professional awareness of it.

Fasting is generally defined as the systematic, voluntary abstention from taking solid food, (and liquids that contain proteins or fats) for 24 hours or more, which is approximately how long it takes ingested matter to be processed through us. When the supply is not replenished, the body begins a series of internal physical responses and metabolic changes that are inherently cleansing and repairing.

Not eating allows the organs to empty and rest, conserving energy, promoting the elimination of waste and accumulated toxins, and making new cell regeneration much more efficient. It may even extend life: Laboratory studies show that rats that are systematically fasted consistently live longer than those fed daily.[1]

Given the nomadic, survival-oriented lifestyle of our primitive ancestors, the periodic lack of food must have been a regular part of the human experience for millennia. During 99% of our history as a species (i.e., the millions of years before the advent of a stable agriculture), the empty-full digestion cycle was a regular condition of life, undoubtedly influencing our evolution. Notwithstanding our recent, Western habit of being perpetually satiated (if not completely stuffed !), fasting—the periodic resting of the gastro-intestinal organs—is a natural human activity.

The relatively new phenomenon of an over-abundant food supply has spelled the end of the truly ecological regulation of our eating habits. We've gained this easy access to food at the expense of much of our health. Today, 40% of all Americans are overweight,[2] and overeating has become an epidemic of chronic substance-abuse and self-destruction. It is one of the most prevalent health-endangering behaviors in our society.

Among the debilitating effects of long-term over-eating and poor diet, which fasting aims at correcting, is intestinal blockage. This occurs when the efficiency of our waste-removal system is impaired by too much food, a lack of fibre, and insufficient physical activity. The results are compaction, diverticulum (intestinal pockets of accumulated waste), and constipation. These in turn lead to poor assimilation of nutrients, the starvation of cells, and an accumulation of bacteria that can eventually cause autotoxemia, a slow self-poisoning. Naturopaths and internal hygienists, the traditional champions of fasting and its adjunct therapy, colonic irrigation, contend that these conditions of internal pollution are the origin of many common health problems. They point out that *we are not nourished by the amount of food we eat, but by the amount we can properly assimilate.* Often eating at all actually complicates sickness.

Fasting is a viable alternative to the expensive and risk-prone pharmacological approach. If we were taught to consult our own body-wisdom as readily as we do medicine men, we would discover that, in most cases, the system needs less, not more. Indeed, we merely have to observe the fasting behavior of ailing animals in the wild to verify the natural wisdom of giving the digestive system a rest during healing. The common experience of "losing your appetite" when sick may be nature's call to fast.

(Day 1)—My reasons for fasting: Feeling sluggish. Joints are creaky. I need a general renewal of energy for upcoming projects. Plus, like most Americans, I'm a borderline food abuser. This fast should help me exercise better judgement in self-care. If nothing else, I'll save some money not eating! I feel both eager and apprehensive. Getting nostalgic about the refrigerator!

Fasting may be the most ancient healing strategy known to man. Its under-utilization in our culture seems puzzling, in view of its long history and world-wide acceptance in both religious and healing contexts. In many traditional cultures, including Mediterranean, Oriental, East Indian, and Native American, it has been regarded as among the most dependable curative and revitalizing personal health measures.

Christ was not being metaphoric when he said we don't live by bread alone! A third century Aramaic manuscript preserved in the Vatican archives quotes him as giving extensive instruction on how to heal oneself through fasting.[3] The Buddha is said to have survived for months at a time on one grain of rice per day. Other great figures who were noted for their low rate of food consumption include the great Tibetan poet/yogi, Milarepa, and the Indian holy man, Shiva Puri Baba, who lived 140 years.[4]

Hippocrates prescribed fasting, as did Galen and Paracelsus, and it was practiced by Plato, Socrates, Pythagoras, and Mahatma Gandhi. Even today, in Europe, reputable clinics and doctors that support therapeutic fasting are quite common. In Sweden it's practically a national sport, as accepted as jogging and aerobics are in the United States.[5]

Can (or should) fasting be used as a therapeutic intervention for specific ailments? It depends on who you ask. The debate is drawn along the line between clinical and anecdotal evidence. One side, primarily the stand of medical scientists, points to the lack of controlled, statistical research on the efficacy of therapeutic fasting. To them, technically acceptable proof would require double-blind studies of separate fasting and non-fasting groups with the same illnesses, a research task that's never been attempted, probably because those most involved in supervised fasting are more interested in individuals than statistics.

This lack of data unfortunately leads to many misconceptions about fasting, and tends to prevent its more general use. What information the scientists do rely on comes from the study of numerous cases of people starving under extremely adverse conditions: prisoners of war, political protesters, institutionalized schizophrenics, etc. Most of these studies are attempts to chart the abnormal metabolic effects of forced starvation, and the progressive physical deterioration which, if unchecked, can lead to death.[6] Within this clinical setting, only two medical conditions have been accepted as possible indications for fasting—extreme obesity and schizophrenia—and then only as a last resort.[7]

The general view of this camp is well summed-up by nutritionist/biochemist Marion Nestle, Ph.D. at the University of California Medical School, San Francisco, and nutrition advisor to *Medical Self Care* magazine: "Healthy people can fast for up to two weeks with no harm. The real question is whether it does any good. I don't know of any studies that show that not eating is better than good nutrition. Someone who is ill should not fast, because it's going to make them worse. My own approach is that food is great and people ought to eat it."

Even more opposed to fasting is nutritionist and author of *Get Well Naturally* Linda Clark, who refers to a study (by four physicians at the University of California Department of Medicine and School of Public Health, L.A.) of eleven obese patients who maintained a prolonged fast on water and vitamin pills. "Serious complications developed in every one of the cases, including temporary anemia, low blood pressure, and gout. The problems usually disappeared after the patients began to eat again." The conclusion of the study: Prolonged fasting is hazardous.[8]

Clark also feels that the would-be detoxifying action of fasting leads to a uniquely modern problem: Poisonous accumulated toxins, such as DDT, which are stored in human fat tissue, are released into the blood stream during the fast. She feels this is reason enough to warn us against fasting.[9]

And a recent article in *Prevention* magazine quotes Harvard Medical School professor George Blackburn, M.D., Ph.D., as saying, "There are no known therapeutic reasons for a total fast . . . ," warning that protein, mineral and fluid losses during fasting "could lead to heart attack or stroke."[10]

But the proponents of fasting offer reams of testimonials from recovered arthritics, asthmatics, hypertensives, insomniacs, and ex-victims of migraines, skin and digestive disorders, and dozens of other ailments. (See section below, Ailments Commonly Helped by Therapeutic Fasting) At one famous clinic in Germany, Otto H.F. Buchinger, whom nutritionalist Paavo Airola calls "the world's greatest authority on fasting," has over the past fifty years supervised over 70,000 therapeutic fasts, many lasting months, with virtually no dangerous or serious after-effects.[11] In the U.S., Dr. Bernard Jensen, author of *Tissue Cleansing Through Bowel Management* has supervised over 50,000 fasts at his center in Escondido, California.

Fasting advocates object to the way medical scientists often use the words *fasting* and *starvation* interchangeably. Clearly the difference between carefully conducted therapeutic fasts and the clinical examples of high-stress starvation *in extremis* is an important, if contextual one. Experienced advocates maintain that, with the important exception of a few serious diseases (see Contra-indications), the systematic voluntary abstention from food, under positive, supportive conditions, is almost always a healthy response to illness and, because of its preventive influence, more so as *an early*, not last resort. This amounts to a controlled detoxification, conservation of energy for healing, and the efficient regeneration of new tissue. Real starvation, by this definition, occurs only long after abstention from food begins, when essential nutrients are no longer available from stored and recycled sources within the body and the break-down of vital, healthy tissue ensues. At that point, genuine hunger returns and signals the need for solid food, well in advance of the time that damage to the system would occur.

The problems of mineral loss and the release of toxins into the bloodstream highlight an important distinction in methods of fasting. The old style "total fast" (or "water fast") allows no nutritional liquids. Its advocates maintain that it induces the most complete internal purification,[12] but it is also the most shocking to the system. Dr. Rudolph Ballentine, M.D., author of *Diet & Nutrition—a Holistic Approach*, and physician at the Himalayan International Institute (Honesdale, Penn.), points out that unlike fasters of other times, whose fat reserves contained the whole spectrum of essential nutrients necessary to sustain life in lean times, the average American today has no such stores, given the gross deficiencies of our typical fare. This makes water fasting a greater risk in modern times.[13]

The safer and more gradual "juice fast" uses natural vegetable and fruit juices to provide essential vitamins to sustain metabolism, and minerals which neutralize toxins released in the body and help the system remove pollutants.[14] It is the juice fast which is most utilized in European clinics and American health resorts, and the method most often used today for therapeutic application. (Unfortunately, it is the fasting procedure least studied by research scientists.) Airola and others argue that supplying valuable, easily assimilated vitamins, minerals, enzymes, electrolytes, and trace elements through fresh vegetable juices and broths does not interfere with the resting of the digestive system (the nutritious liquids are absorbed directly into the blood stream from the upper tract) or the elimination of metabolic waste. But this type of fasting does safeguard against serious deficiencies. The juices also provide an alkalizing influence, balancing the acidification of the system which fasting induces.[15]

Doctors at The Sacramento Preventive Medicine Clinic have supervised thousands of therapeutic fasts since first observing its remarkable effect on one patient's "terminal" intestinal cancer. After a 21-day therapeutic fast, "the radiologist swore that it couldn't be the same man," reports Dr. Michael Kwiker, an osteopath with the clinic. Six years later, he remains in excellent health.

Ironically, the clinic does not take patients with cancer, nor advise them to fast, for reasons that are more sociopolitical than medical: Alternative therapies are under heavy scrutiny in California these days. The team of doctors at the Sacramento clinic utilizes the "elimination diet" and "bowel cleansing" only with the less life-threatening illnesses, and only after all other therapies have been tried. Still, Dr. Kwiker believes that "fasting is one of the safest, lowest-risk forms of therapy." Americans, he says, "haven't begun to appreciate the fact that the body really does need to clean out. When it's done with intelligent supervision and a sense of understanding, fasting is extremely safe." The clinic maintains a full-time hotline for fasting out-patients and offers public lectures on internal hygiene every Tuesday evening.[16]

Dr. Kwiker, who fasts about twice a year because he "likes the feeling," says he cannot think of a single case in which fasting hasn't benefited the patient. Even in the rare instances when fasts were prematurely terminated (usually for reasons of personal or domestic instability), no harmful effects have ever been observed.

Dr. Kwiker's favorite example of a healthy faster is Mr. V. E.

Irons of Grassville, California. Mr. Irons is a successful business man and well-known lecturer and author. He has been practicing therapeutic and preventive fasting for over 40 years and is the originator of the fasting protocol used at the Sacramento Preventive Medicine clinic. At 91 he has a 14 year-old son, an 18 year-old daughter, and a 66 year old son! Mr. Irons lectures regularly in California on bowel cleansing. People are continuously astounded at how young and healthy he looks.

AILMENTS COMMONLY HELPED BY THERAPEUTIC FASTING

As a healing intervention, fasting is reported—in anecdotal literature and at fasting centers—to be most beneficial in cases of stress syndromes, chronic functional disorders, and systemic imbalances, as opposed to acute organ failure, structural breakdown, infectious diseases, or similar emergency conditions. Fasting is good for:

- Digestive & eliminative disorders: constipation, diarrhea, colitis, gas, etc.
- Arthritis, rheumatism, bursitis.
- High blood pressure.
- Asthma, emphysema, chronic bronchitis.
- Glandular imbalances.
- Overweight & underweight.
- Edema.
- Toxemia & related problems: dermatitis, eczema, halitosis.
- Sinusitis.
- Weak immune system: low grade infections, colds.
- Chronic allergies, hay fever.
- Chronic headaches.
- Some forms of heart disease & impaired circulation.

(Day 3)—Blood pressure and pulse down. Not really hungry, but missing tastes and chewing. Having olfactory hallucinations of cooking odors! Very aware of my body: senses, heartbeat, energy, etc. After enema: headache gone, energy returned. Tends to confirm

intestinal auto-toxemia theory. Very empowering feeling, like my first fast when arthritis began to clear up. What a gift!

How does the body get the elements vital to metabolism while the intestines are empty? It is true that protein is initially taken from muscle and other tissue, but this "autolysis" breaks down and burns body cells in inverse order of importance (excess, old, weak and diseased matter is taken first)[17] and actually recycles the amino acids, the building blocks of protein. This explains how blood protein (serum albumin levels) can remain stable, and how "anabolism," the synthesis of new cells, can take place during fasting. In this way, says Airola, nature in her wisdom protects the vital organs, glands, nervous system and brain from deterioration well into the second *month* of fasting.[18].

After a few days, and increasingly thereafter, the fats stored in adipose tissue and the liver break down and release stored carbohydrates, glucose, ketones, and other fuels for energy.[19] (The reduction of body insulation makes it important to stay warm during fasting.) On the average, weight loss will be between one and two pounds per day.

When the fat supply is exhausted, the body will resort to taking protein from healthy muscle tissue, and deterioration/starvation will commence. But this is the point at which a true, strong hunger returns, nature's signal that the therapeutic stage has ended, and so should the fast.

During a fast, uric acid, purines, and the acidic by-products of fat metabolism enter the blood stream. This "acidosis" is one reason why systemic blood and lymph diseases, such as anemia, leukemia, and gout are on the list of contra-indications for fasting. But fasting authorities maintain that in most cases such transient toxicosis is a natural healing response (like running a fever) and recommend the alkalinity of fruit and vegetable juices to offset acidity, mediate changes in blood volume, and insure the excretion of unwanted poisons through the urine.[20] Dr. Kwiker teaches his patients to self-monitor their urine acidity with paper test strips, and points out that encouraging regular kidney and bowel functions with vegetable broths usually prevents acid build-up.

At Northeast Community Hospital, in Bedford, Texas, clinical ecologist Dr. Stevan Cordas sometimes administers implants of alkalizing salts, such as baking soda, to neutralize acidity in his fasting patients. "We expect adverse reactions," says Dr. Cordas. "Those who need it the most have a re-creation of their symptoms." For this reason, he is among those who caution against fasting at home.

Past president of the International Academy of Preventive Medicine, Dr. Cordas has supervised over 1700 fasts in a highly-controlled, ultra-hygienic clinical environment in order to isolate allergens, and micro-toxic foods and pollutants that cause life-long non-specific debilitaing syndromes. This unique method of diagnostic fasting has led to the startling conclusion that 80% of all migraine headaches and 30% of all asthma attacks are precipitated by such offensive stimulants.[21]

(Day 5)—Mouth still feels very pastey. Body chills gone, even though it's a colder day. I'm convinced this is adding years to my life. This is real life insurance! Dinner: hot carrot/beet juice. Delicious. Solid food seems strangely foreign.

What other side effects can be expected from fasting? Sensations of queasiness and even nausea may appear within the first 48 hours, as the stomach, intestines and digestive organs adjust to the novel situation of going off-cycle, emptying and shrinking. Loss of energy and possibly mild headache may signal the temporary re-absorption of decayed matter, loosened from intestinal walls. With sufficient fluid intake, these signs usually disappear within a day.

Since fasting activates all the organs and systems of elimination (skin, lungs, liver, kidneys, bowels, sinuses, and the lymph system), initial side-effects will often include bad breath, coated tongue, mucous discharge, complexion erup-tions, dandruff, dark and odorous urine and stools, and other purification responses, depending upon the degree of pollution built up in the system prior to fasting. Unfortunately, the uninformed will respond with alarm to these admittedly unpleasant experiences, although they are actually positive signs that a much-needed, albeit accelerated, housecleaning has begun. It may even trigger a "healing crisis," manifesting symptoms of old illnesses that were suppressed with drugs. It is at such times that foreknowledge of expected effects, good supervision, and support are most helpful.

It is always preferable to plan a fast with the advice and consent of your own physician, but an M.D. who has no familiarity with fasting as a therapy (which describes the vast majority of American doctors) may not support your fast for that reason alone and not necessarily because it won't be good for you. Therefore, what you learn from alternative sources, including books, experienced fasters, and your own body/intuition may be as valid as the opinon of an uninformed allopath. In general, it's safe to say that if you are in reasonably good health, you are qualified to try at least a short fast of a few days duration. When in doubt, the novice faster should begin to take light, nourishing foods and try to learn what the body is saying.

CONTRA-INDICATIONS

Certain acute conditions are not compatible with fasting. These include: tuberculosis, highly infectious diseases, bleeding ulcers, advanced or juvenile diabetes, hypoglycemia, gout, blood, liver and kidney diseases, active malignancies, coronary thrombosis and myocardial infarctions. In addition, fasting is contra-indicated in conditions of emaciation and pregnancy (although one writer contends that "morning sickness," with its concomitant loss of appetite, is nature's way of purifying the system for childbearing[22]). People on medications are likewise not advised to fast. The personality types that should not fast include compulsive/addictives and those that suffer from anorexia nervosa and/or bulimia.

HOW TO FAST

The first part of fasting is education. It is essential that the candidate be able to conduct the fast properly, and there are several important rules which will help insure safety and success.

The timing of a fast is important. Ideally, it is not undertaken at a time of unusual stress. Although abstaining from food is often not as difficult as the novice may imagine, it is useful to plan ahead. In particular, during the first two days, when you may feel weak and out of sorts, it's nice to be able to be alone, or with supportive loved ones, in a peaceful setting, and to rest (and sleep) when you feel like it. If necessary, enlist the cooperation of friends and family so that they will not weaken your resolve with ridicule and temptations.

One should begin to taper off in quantity and complexity of diet several days before all solid food is eliminated. This reduces the mental and physical shock of not eating. While fasting, generous amounts of liquid (at least two quarts per day) should be taken to internally wash the system of accumulated toxins and waste. For the same reason, many authorities recommend high enemas once a day. Airola and others maintain that, given the obstructed and toxic state of the intestines of most Americans by middle age, it would be dangerous to fast without enemas. A professional colonic irrigation in mid-fast greatly augments the internal cleansing process.

Note that a fast will only be hygienically and therapeutically effective if the liquids consumed contain no proteins or fats, so that the body will begin to break down its own excess and polluted tissue. Milk is out. Herbal teas and hot, clear broths are allowed. Juices for fasting can be made from carrots, cucumbers, celery, beets, greens, peppers, and berries, as well as most fruits. Dr. Cordas especially recommends cabbage juice for its high enzyme and vitamin content. An electric vegetable juicer is a great asset for fasting, assuring the freshest possible nutrients at the time of injection. In all cases, the liquids used should be as pure and fresh as possible. If organically-grown produce is unavailable, vegetables and fruit should be thoroughly washed before juicing. It's fun to discover the art of the liquid lunch!

In addition, some people take certain natural substances for specific healing effects while fasting: Psyllium seeds are a natural laxative; chlorophyll, lemon juice, and beet tablets are traditional liver cleansers; Bentonite (volcanic ash) absorbs poisons; potato water is high in Vitamin C; and garlic kills bacteria and viruses. (Garlic Tonic: Put 1/2 clove into the vegetable juicer, then juice vegetables through the garlic pulp. Enjoy!)

The difference in opinions between "experts" points to the need for intelligent discrimination in choosing a fasting strategy. As with many other health philosophies, fasting has its fanatic fringe, inclined to making wild and excessive claims, and giving a dubious reputation to an otherwise sound theory. This is just another reason to consult a wide variety of sources and weigh the evidence carefully. Beware, for example, of the mono-vegie fasts which recommend unusual amounts of only one kind of juice.

(Day 6)—To say that I'm sleeping well would be an understatement—this is really profound! Very vivid, memorable dreams. Feeling good. Gave three massages today with no problem. Lost weight, gained energy. Lunch: onion-parsley tea. Yum.

Among possible early food-withdrawal symptoms is a mild mental depression, as habitual oral gratification and the social reinforcements associated with dinner-times are withheld. Unfulfilled attachments to particularly addictive "foods" such as sugar, coffee, etc. may manifest as emotional mood swings. (It's uncanny how unusually tempting foods will seem to appear to test your discipline!) Fasting has a way of highlighting such issues as personal purpose, commitment, and freedom. Fasting can be emotionally as well as physically catalytic. Prepare yourself and those you live with for these symptoms. Invariably, initial difficulties are replaced by a satisfied feeling of accomplishment as attachments and desires are overcome. Paradoxically, the longer you fast, the less hungry you feel.

It may be helpful to write down your own list of reasons for fasting, and review them from time to time. Keep a journal of your thoughts, feelings, and insights. Fasting is very much a process of self-discovery. It entails exploring one's psycho-spiritual aspects as well as physical. Meditation and prayer are very appropriate to this process.

The fourteenth century Islamic poet and mystic, Al-Ghazzali recommended fasting as "the only act of worship which is not seen by anyone except God." It gives one a sense of freedom, not only from the weight and discomfort of an overburdened and inefficient system, but from the tyranny of one's old habits and desires. It's a new kind of freedom of choice, action, and timing. As a self-administered therapy, it helps promote confidence, autonomy, and personal power. It engenders a heightened sense of clarity, well being, and enthusiasm, due partially to more efficient metabolism, and partially to the sense of accomplishment it affords.

Aside from the psychological high of self-mastery, the mild euphoria often reported by fasters around the third day may be traced to the same neurochemical changes that athletes undergo when getting their "second wind," as endorphins and peptides are released in the brain.[23] Dr. Kwiker also explains that fat digestion, which only commences after available sugars and carbohydrates are burned, provides a more steady and strong metabolic functioning, which predictably translates into feelings of heightened personal power. (He suggests curbing one's enthusiasm and resisting temptations to embark on any herculean tasks at this time!)

Nevertheless, regular moderate exercise during the fast is not only permissible, but beneficial to maintain good circulation and elimination. Yoga is an excellent adjunct practice, as are breathing exercises and inversions. So is swimming. The value of fresh air, pure water, and sunlight during this purification process cannot be over-emphasized. Since the skin is the single largest organ of elimination, dry brush massage and warm baths are also co-therapeutic.

One way to maximize the elimination of deposited waste material from the intestinal tract, and tonify the digestive organs, is to practice deep self-massage of the abdominal cavity. This entails relaxing the related abdominal muscles, and slowly and gently probing the inner organs in a circular motion. Mild discomfort may mean that the system is "backed-up" or gaseous. This should disappear within 24 hours. Any acute pain during self-massage indicates a trip to the doctor is in order.

Older people, pregnant women, and people with major digestive or colonic impairments should consult their physician before any deep manipulation. Contra-indications would include active ulcers, malignancies, diverticulitis, aneurysms (ballooned blood vessels), and embolisms (blood clots).

(Day 8)—Cut and stacked 1/2 cord of firewood, but endurance is lower than normal. Looks like my posture has improved. Joints pain-free. Had the feeling my body was giving thanks for the opportunity to be so light and clean. Dreamt of baklava!

BREAKING THE FAST

To empty the gastro-intestinal tract, and commence autolysis and the breakdown of excess adipose tissue, a biologically therapeutic fast must last at least three days. How much longer one can or should fast depends upon such factors as age, medical condition, extent of toxification, body weight, lifestyle, reactions, and other individual factors. The average length of fasts at most health spas in Europe is between ten and twenty days, but fasts twice as long are not uncommon. The longest recorded controlled therapeutic fast lasted 382 days.[24] In many cases, fasts are repeated in cycles, interspersed with periods of taking light, natural foods, usually exclusively vegetarian. For fasts over ten days long, experienced supervision is recommended.

Setting a goal for the length of the fast can be helpful, but it's best not to be rigid or overly programed. Consult your intuition and your body, as well as your schedule, about continuing. Regularly re-assess your condition and be intelligently flexible.

In many ways, breaking the fast is the most critical phase. Because the system has been at rest, and the organs have shrunk, and because human nature can be impetuous, the first few days after a fast should be conducted with the utmost care. Not uncommonly, taking only the appropriate amounts of food after fasting calls for more will power and control than not eating at all. One good rule of thumb is to re-introduce solid foods over the course of as many days as the fast itself lasted. If you get into a "back to normal" rate of food consumption too soon, you are liable to tax your system and do more damage than if you had never fasted. *Break the fast gradually*, with small amounts of wholesome foods such as fresh salad vegetables. Plan meals carefully and keep portions modest. Chew thoroughly (Digestion begins with mastication. "Drink your food.") Know how to stop, and leave the table well *before saturation*, for the tendency is to congratulate oneself, relax one's vigilance, and over-do it. Be wise.

The end of a fast offers an excellent opportunity to study the effects of specific foods on the system. The mono-substance approach to re-entry is particularly useful for allergy diagnosis, allowing isolation of the offending food-allergen. Any adverse reactions are immediately noticeable in contrast to the general feeling of well-being attained by the fast. Conversely, some very nutritious foods may make you feel exceptionally good as their energy is released in the body.

Obviously, the choice of diet following a fast will greatly affect how lasting its benefits may be. Fasting, like eating well, and all self-care measures, teaches us one valuable lesson: You may not know if you can do it, but you can be sure nobody else can do it for you! Good Luck.

(Day 10)—Cooking is a much more conscious experience. I feel more intuitive in the kitchen. As for the eating, my born-again taste buds are dancing with joy! Fresh garden vegie-soup: Bits of carrots, peppers, beets, parsley, tomatoes, with a dash of soy sauce and dark sesame oil. Ah . . . Feel like I'm glowing all over. Who would have thought self-denial would be such a high!

ONE PERSON'S INTRODUCTION TO FASTING

I first tried therapeutic fasting when, in my 28th year, I was suddenly stricken with a painful case of rheumatoid arthritis. My shoulder ached, my left knee was swollen stiff, and my wrists and hands were so sore I lost a landscaping job because I could no longer push a lawn mower. My life had come to an abrupt and painful impasse.

A rheumatologist extracted nearly a cup of dark green fluid from my stricken knee. After more than $300 worth of tests, I was informed that there was no known cure for my condition. To ease the pain in my joints, I was told to take a dozen aspirin a day and watch for signs of internal hemorrhaging. My search for alternatives began.

I asked everyone I met what they knew about arthritis. I haunted health food stores, libraries, and bookstores. My search led me to Paavo Airola's book, *There Is a Cure for Arthritis*. The cure was internal cleanliness, and fasting was one of the main methods.

My first few fasts were only three days long, but they were great learning experiences, and I was surprised to discover that not eating was easier than I had anticipated. I loved the new-found feeling of being empty, and noticed immediate improvements in my energy level and experience of sleep.

Most gratifying, however, was the gradual diminishing of my joint pains over the course of the next four months. While it would be impossible to ascribe my recovery to fasting alone (since I engaged in a comprehensive, multi-therapy program which also included dietary restrictions, nutritional supplements, herbal remedies, yoga, and massage), I have no doubt that the fasts helped heal my joints. I never took the aspirins, and soon my painful handicap was a memory.

Over the eleven years since that first fast, I've used fasting to clear up a case of colitis, heal some enlarged hemorhoids, eliminate headaches and other minor symptoms, and increase my energy. I've concluded that—for me—systematic under-eating and periodic fasting are good health strategies. I feel best with basically one main meal per day. I like to fast a few days a year, and have tried various timing intervals: on solstice days, monthy, and—Mahatma Gandhi's method—the weekly fast. Cyclical or seasonal fasting puts one strongly in touch with the basic and universal elements of nature, and renews our respect for the precious and endangered chain of life. Some feel that the experience of this connection alone is worth the effort of fasting.

I have several good friends with a few years' experience in fasting, all positive. One lived perfectly healthfully and otherwise quite normally on vegetable juices alone for 45 days, for spiritual reasons. Indeed it was from observing her that I realized that fasting is really no big deal. As a health counselor, I've also had occasion to coach some others who chose this method of self-healing. My role has been to give people all the information I've accumulated on the subject, encourage them to exercise their best judgement, and support them in their self-care process. In the dozen cases I've been involved with, none resulted in any adverse side-effects, while at least one, a fellow arthritis sufferer, showed dramatic improvement.

PROFESSIONAL SUPPORT FOR FASTING

As self-care and person-oriented health philosophies begin to influence the medical profession, more doctors supportive of fasting are becoming available. Some two dozen such practitioners are listed in *The National Directory of Holistic Health Professionals* (Association for Holistic Health, P.O. Box 9532, San Diego, CA 92109) Another directory can be found in Bernard Jensen's *Tissue Cleansing Through Bowel Management.* And the International Academy of Biological Medicine

(P.O. Box 31313, Phoenix, AZ 85046), founded by fasting advocate/nutritionist Paavo Airola, also distributes a directory of members. The Society of Clinical Ecology (2005 Franklin St., Suite 490, Denver, CO 80205) can put you in touch with hospital-based fasting programs in several major cities. You may also want to show this chapter to your own family physician to see if he or she would support your fast.

Two natural health organizations that offer information about therapeutic fasting are: The International Naturopathic Association (874 North Beverly Glen Blvd., Los Angeles, CA 90077), and the American Natural Hygiene Society, Inc. (698 Brooklawn Ave., Bridgeport, CT 06604).

In addition, several alternative health centers around the country support therapeutic juice fasting, bowel cleansing, and purification diets. The Sacramento Preventive Medical Group, mentioned above, is at 1816 Tribute Rd., Sacramento, CA 95815. Hippocrates Health Institute (25 Exeter St., Boston, MA 02116), founded by nutritionist Ann Wigmore, emphasizes the use of the juices of wheat grass and other sprouted, live vegetable foods. Dr. Bernard Jensen's Hidden Valley Health Ranch is at Rt. 1, Box 52, Escondido, CA 92025.

One of the most well-established residential health centers supporting fasting is Meadowlark (26126 Fairview Ave., Hemet, CA 92344). Founded by Dr. Evarts Loomis twenty-five years ago, the center offers medically supervised healing regimes that also include exercise, relaxation, and a thorough and eclectic self-health care educational program, all in an idyllic country setting. The average fast lasts between one and two weeks.

An excellent East Coast equivalent is Turnwood Organic Gardens (Livingston Manor, NY 12758). Not a medical facility, Turnwood is staffed by a team of holistic nutritionists who offer personally-tailored organic juice programs, exercise and stress reduction techniques, complete recreational and sports facilities, and a natural health library. Lectures on addiction and weight loss, juice fasting, sprouting, and vegetarianism, and workshops on such self-care strategies as yoga and meditation, are built into the program. Guests are continuously monitored, in consultation with their own physicians if necessary. Chiropractic and massage treatments are also available. Turnwood's thoughtful brochure is an education in itself.

Lastly, taped lectures and classes on fasting, by some of the leading contemporary experts, are available from Natural Hygiene Press (12816 Race Track Road, Tampa, FL 33625).

HOW I USE FASTING

The following is my personal list of reasons for fasting. Notice that only the first is "Healing." I find it useful to refer to this list when my resolve wavers during a fast. The list continues to grow.

- Healing. Prevention. Immunological resistance. Optimum systemic resiliency.
- General good feelings. Joy, lightness, personal accomplishment. A natural high.
- Body cleaning. Metabolic efficiency. Internal detoxification, waste removal, purification.
- Increased mental alertness. Subtle refinement of awareness. Mindfulness, concentration, perception, sensitivity, discrimination, judgment. ESP.
- Greater vitality, energy. Productivity, creativity, perseverance.
- Freedom from compulsiveness and slavery to appetite.
- Spiritual discipline, meditation. Calmness, peace of mind. Mediates stress.
- Sleep less. Breathe easier. Live longer.
- Better yoga and sports performance.
- Self-massage of inner organs.
- Save money, save time.
- Detachment as practice for easier dying.
- Ecological/social conscience. Third-World awareness.
- Heightened body/sensory awareness.
- Work with personal issues and dynamics: values, priorities, attachment, desire, judgement, commitment.
- Developing personal strength of character/confidence.

~°~°~°~

V.

THE SPIRIT OF HEALING

... illness is the result of holding a wrong philosophy, one which permits one to behave foolishly and disharmoniously, one which does not help one to perceive the body and the mind as a whole. The right philosophy, on the other hand, must aid one in the quest for deeper meaning, which in turn is a constituent of our overall wholeness ... cosmology is relevant for correct thinking and good health ... to be whole is to be encompassed by the sense of the divine cosmos.
                                                    —Henry Skolimowski

THE STRESS OF SELF-CENTEREDNESS

Some people seem to move gracefully through life's changes, confident in the knowledge of their basic connection with the world. They feel at home in the universe. For these peaceful souls, everything is a gift or a teaching. All problems are temporary. These folks laugh a lot. They are the lights among us. They have, we would say, a healthy outlook on life.

But many more people in our society feel no such sense of belonging or support. Most seem to be living under the permanent unconscious assumption that they can only survive by somehow "holding it all together," and maintaining control. Keep a stiff upper lip. Watch out. All too often, life seems like more suffering than it's worth. Instead of finding "the Kingdom Within," too many people are fighting for a little space in a hard and hostile environment; behaving as if they'll lose everything if they really relax. Trust is a nice idea, but rarely a direct body/mind experience. For the most part, we are far from "the lilies of the field."

Furthermore, most of us usually seem to be vaguely on our way to somewhere, to do something important in the future. We have lost the ability to be comfortable in the here and now. We are so involved in doing things, we have forgotten what it means to just *be*. In short, we are usually in a state of chronic, non-specific, anxious tension. Even in sleep—nature's time for rest and regeneration—complete peace eludes many, so ingrained are the defenses in the body, so unsettled the mind.

Missing is the contemplative moment, the grace of letting one's mind transcend the personal and the petty, to find a more spacious sense of existence. Absent is the simple gift of serenity, that full, refreshing respite from our driving ambitions and compelling fears, which truly soothes the soul. Few people know how to stop pushing themselves and coast in the energy-conserving mode of "mental neutral." Without ever touching this inner calm, life can become a humorless and exhausting grind.

This contracted way of life often translates into chronic muscle tension. People are literally "uptight." Reichian therapists call it "body armour." Typical dysfunctional consequences of chronic "holding on" include muscle spasm, back pain, high blood pressure, digestive disorders, hemorrhoids, tension and migraine headaches, insomnia and exhaustion. In the extreme, negative feelings of anger and hostility have been linked with heart disease and clogged arteries. This same tense, defensive/offensive way of relating to life is an exacerbating factor in asthma, arthritis, and many other systemic and organ stress disorders.

Why do so many people push themselves so hard and treat themselves so poorly as to self-induce these conditions? What overriding factors enable human beings to continue to engage in such unhealthy, counter-productive, self-defeating behavior? Two main reasons seem to be fear and obsessive ambition: Life is a chronic battle because we are either perpetually protecting ourselves, or trying to get something we don't have. Constantly subjected to the push of our anxieties, and the pull of passion, we are running to something, or from something all the time. In socio-biological terms, this dynamic is called "Fight or Flight."

Fear and ambition are related, and therein lies a clue to the cure for the modern condition. The common denominator in the negative states of fear, greed, jealousy, and hatred is the problem of a distorted sense of self, and an undeveloped sense of connection to the greater whole. The mirror syndromes of superiority and inferiority complexes both stem from the same mis-identification with an isolated identity. Whether we feel small and paranoid, or the Lord of the Universe, with all the stress attached to either position, the problem is the same: the exclusive identification with, and attention to the self, and the subsequent false needs of defense and consumption.

These dynamics often directly translate into the behavior illnesses of over-compensation or over-achievement: obsessive time compulsion, "Type A behavior," social alienation, anxiety attacks, and substance abuse. The inevitable results are the illnesses of chronic exhaustion, and the thousand symptoms that a modern citizen is heir to. These are not *diseases* in the classical sense. They are behavioral illnesses stemming from what the Buddhists call "wrong view," a dysfunctional outlook on the world that severs a person's connection to the Whole.

Predictably, conventional allopathic medicine offers little in the way of real cure for spiritually based sickness. Typically, it provides chemical amelioration for pain and other unpleasant symptoms. Even many of the popular stress-reduction techniques only smooth the surface of the malaise, and never touch the fundamental problem.

To be truly healed, we must eliminate the primary underlying condition supporting and perpetuating chronic stress. I believe this to be the primitive fear-stance towards life (and death), which comes from a fundamental, un-examined, and erroneous psychological assumption about oneself, and the world: namely, that *I am separate from the rest of creation.* I am convinced that the egocentric identification with a small, temporary and vulnerable body/personality, and the resultant state of perpetual self-protection, is the root cause not only of much mental dis-ease and many of our physical afflictions, but our social ills as well.

Physician/psychiatrist, George Hogben, in his essay, "Spiritual Awareness as a Healing Process," states the problem in theological terms. If the word "God" gets in the way, try substituting "The Universe":

Many sick people I have seen do not have an intimate relationship with God. They do not believe that God is in them through each breath they take, waking or sleeping, working or recreating, even during the most mundane activities. They do not sense the Spirit working within them. Even sick people who are strongly religious may be empty of Spirit because for them God is "up there" until the next life. They do not experience the movement of God now!... The internal state is characterized by an essential lifelessness at the core of the individual's being. It is as if a light or primary energy has been extinguished. The consciousness that develops under this condition is one of scarcity, isolation, ego-centricity, and meaning restricted to the transitory and material. This kind of consciousness spawns a social ethic of closed communication and no-holds-barred competitiveness. It generates effects of fear and anxiety, guilt, anger, and rage.[1]

SPIRITUAL STRESS REDUCTION
It is essential that self-image be transformed in healing.
—George Hogben

In Buddhist medicine, all illness is seen as stemming from ignorance, fear, and craving. These are the three "poisons" that are the source of all suffering. The first gives rise to the other two. "Ignorance" (pali: *avijja*) means ignorance of the emptiness of the illusion of self (pali: *anatta*: no self; empty of self-abidingness). This doctrine maintains that who we think we are is in actuality nothing more than a conceptual invention, a convenient illusion, based on the *apparent* solidity and cohesion of body and personality. It is the protection of this false self, and the pursuit of its manufactured needs, which gives rise to fear, grasping, anger, and the ten thousand distresses of an imbalanced, uncontrolled life. Meditation is medicine because it allows us to see through the illusion we're fighting to hold together. Enlightenment is good for your health.

Erich Fromm put it this way:

Well-being is possible only to the degree to which one has overcome one's narcissism; to the degree to which one is open, responsive, sensitive, awake, empty... Well-being means to be fully related to man and nature effectively, to overcome separateness and alienation, to arrive at the experience of oneness with all that exists.

We can relax/heal our bodies only when we eliminate the debilitating fear that comes from feeling isolated. All fear and worry is self-perpetuating, self-defeating, and actually without content or justification. It's also bad for your health.

The solution lies in seeing that there is nobody to protect, that the difference between "alone" and "all one" is one of perception. Fundamental healing can occur when we can (at least momentarily) surrender, or see through, our limited definition of ourselves. To be renewed, we must be able to let go of our old identity. Since such an ego-death is not always easy, many (perhaps most) cannot commit themselves to the process, which is why Dr. Bernie Siegel calls those that can, "exceptional."

Gurdjieff said that the most difficult thing to give up is our own suffering. Like the disobedient child who resorts to earning the disapproval of his negligent parents in a desperate attempt to gain *any* recognition at all, the blind ego will assert itself through negativity and self-affliction rather than sur-render its identity. All too easily, we identify with the safe familiarity of our problems. At least they are our own!

To regain health, it is necessary to realize how we unwittingly contribute to, and benefit from sickness. Such "secondary gains" might include the sympathy and support we get when ill; or the long-overdue rest which we can only justify after a total breakdown occurs. From the earliest reinforcement from suddenly concerned parents, to the financial rewards granted by insurance companies, we have learned that getting sick is a permissible means of gaining escape, rest, and care, when "normal" circumstances are unsatisfactory.

This cultural training is insidious and powerful, and requires soul searching and effort to overcome. For many, the pain of disease is the first real motivation to reach a deeper level of honesty with self and world. Notwithstanding the conventional assumptions about illness as enemy, it is seen in the context of spiritual healing as auspicious, because it serves to wake us up to the fragmentation, transgressions and untruth in our lives. Disease is the call for fundamental, creative change which we cannot ignore.

Many cancer survivors have described their illness as fortuitous: an incentive for soul searching, prioritizing of values, and a way of letting some old, dysfunctional aspects of one's self die, while giving birth to others. Often, the disease gives one permission to express long-repressed emotions, and then a greater creativity. To the extent that serious illness forces a confrontation with our habitual assumptions about ourselves and our condition, it is an ally in disguise. We may despair, complain, or panic when confronted with physical pain and loss of control, but every disease is a teacher, goading us on to learn how to live more consciously in our bodies and in the world. Finally, and perhaps even for the first time, the establishment of harmony, internal and external, becomes priority one.

The path to such a transmutation of trouble can seem long and dark. The small self often struggles through the classic stages of dying: denial, anger, bargaining, depression.

We mourn, not only for our lost health, but for our lost self-identity, habits, assumptions, and values. We may have to enter a dark night of the soul before claiming bodily health. We need to learn how to practice mental and spiritual hygiene, as well as physical. Cleansing the soul turns out to be at least as important—and perhaps more difficult—than keeping the body clean.

Seeing illness as opportunity rather than punishment is the first step towards real healing in the psycho-spiritual sense. This is when we stop asking "Why me?" and start asking "Why now?" Hogben calls this *Healing of Consciousness.* The primary medicines are intuition, faith, hope, imagination, forgiveness and love. Others are: compassion, sympathetic joy, and equanimity. Mental, emotional and physical health follow the healing of the soul. Psycho-spiritual healing works because these positive, life affirming sentiments are self-healing, and can be cultivated. One of the easiest ways to assimilate these qualities is to read inspirational literature, itself a kind of placebo, along with religious community and ritual.

HEALING AS RELIGIOUS EXPERIENCE

If you look back, medicine and religion used to be very close together, and what we're trying to do is use a common language—physiology—to show that you can bring the two back together again.   —Herbert Benson, M.D.[2]

My therapeutic goal has more to do with peace of mind than physical healing. Why? Because that is the stuff of which miracles are made.   —Dr. Bernie Siegel, M.D.

Not surprisingly, many people face the personal crisis of illness by relying on their religious faith, especially when their faith in medicine is shaken by poor results. In fact, it may very well be that the *faith itself* is the primary, necessary factor, and the object of faith secondary. Ironically, prayer, affirmations and meditation are sometimes more powerful than drugs, because they affect that ineffable but essential core of the human being, the spirit/soul.

In spite of the fact that there is rarely any reference to their connection in secular schools and hospitals, healing and religion have always been inseparable. In most cultures until recently, including our own, the roles of minister and physician were often one and the same.

People instinctively pray in times of sickness, often with good results. Sociobiologists might account for this by citing the survival value of the metabolic effects of such religious activities as contemplative prayer and meditation, as demonstrated by Benson: All the autonomic parameters of the Relaxation Response change positively. Benson's second book (1984) investigates a second ingredient in the self-healing equation, the "Faith Factor." He has found that relaxation coupled with *belief* gives better ("sometimes remarkable") results than either alone. Clearly, belief systems influence healing, and religious belief systems (cosmologies, paradigms) can influence it dramatically.

But what clinical and statistical studies cannot reveal is the actual *experience* of personal healing. The most important information about "spiritual healing" will always be anecdotal. What makes spiritual/transformational healing so difficult for science to study is that, though it is evidenced by physiological improvement, the real changes are highly subjective. A religiously oriented person has the healing advantage of a (more or less) working relationship to reality at large, call it what they may. He or she can trust the world/universe more readily in difficult times, and this has a healthful influence on the immune, nervous, and cardio-vascular systems.

Another "explanation" for the healing power of prayer might be that it is an exercise in medical imagery. That is, when we "ask" for health, we are actively imagining the possibility of getting it. This moment of positive expectation (in this case prayer-induced) is vital, we might even say *essential,* to the recovery process. To put it another way, try to imagine someone getting well who themselves cannot imagine it! We would say, "They haven't got a prayer!"

THE PSYCHOLOGY OF HOPE

The only common factor that I could find was a change in attitude in the patients prior to "spontaneous remission," a change involving hope and other positive feelings. —Elmer Green[3]

The highly respected researcher, Dr. Lawrence LeShan found hopelessness and helplessness common personality factors in his cancer patients (1977). He describes a particular recurring double bind, in which true self-expression, particularly in lifestyle and livelihood, is perceived to be in direct conflict with an overriding sense of obligation to the wishes and expectations of others.

Each of these cancer patients was in some way living a false or superficial existence, out of the assumption, conscious or otherwise, that to follow their inner calling would cost them their main (often only), significant relationship or life-role. Most often these crippling assumptions about their role in the world were made in early childhood and were associated with traumatic loss.

For these victims, no way out of this conflict was perceived. Psycho-spiritually paralyzed and fatalistic, many were just going through the motions of living their lives as expected. Feeling defeated and doomed, their malignancy actually functioned as a desperate solution to their tormenting stagnation. Time and again, we find that it is the appearance of the disease that catalyzes movement in the patient's life, either towards a new (transformed) existence, or towards the other way out, death. Indeed in some cases, cancer can be seen as a socially acceptable form of suicide.

As a therapist, LeShan's best successes were with patients who could be convinced of the possibility of a "third way" between self-denying conformity on the one hand, and the fear of isolation and failure on the other. His "crisis therapy" is designed to stimulate a strong sense of individual identity and encourage ways to express it. If a patient could rekindle a belief in the possibility of true satisfaction and fulfillment in life, they had a much better chance of survival. LeShan acted as midwife to this necessary sense of hope.

If, in your struggle for greater authenticity and a truer life, in the middle of this spiritual health/identity crisis, you can re-discover a positive connection to the Whole, if you can hear your inner source of inspiration ("guidance," "truth"), and, more than *hear* it, *become* it, you are transformed and so, incidentally, is your body. Everything that has befallen you now has meaning, and you have gained the possibility of completing a *"successful sickness."*

We are saying then, that real healing (as opposed to superficial alleviation or suppression of symptoms) implies, or goes with, a fundamental renewal and transformation of the whole being. By transformation we mean a basic change, not only in external behavior, but also in actual perception of self, world, universe, reality: a paradigmatic shift, which thereafter undeniably alters one's understanding and attitude towards life. Often (but not necessarily), this experience is described in religious terms: Grace. Born again. Slain in the Spirit. Communion. "At-one-ment." It is usually followed by a sense of insight, resolution, and inner peace, even to the extent of losing fear of death itself. In fact, it is a common outcome of clinical Near Death Experiences (NDE). Surgeon/psychiatrist W.E. Ellerbroek, after studying over 60 cases of completely unexpected "spontaneous remissions," concluded that such "miracles" occur only when people are moribund, or prac-tically so. Once again, new life comes from the surrender of the old. The phoenix of regenerated spirit arises from the ashes of the dead ego.

Other psycho-emotional signs of transformation include feelings of renewal, hope, optimism, joy, gratitude, great patience, forgiveness (including self-forgiveness), generosity, and love. Virtually all the cases of cancer remission in the early Simonton programs reported this phenomenon. That is, *there was 100% correlation of remission with self-reported transformation.* (Achterberg, Simonton, & Simonton 1976.)

When we are fully realized under the term "human," transcendent experiences should, in theory, be common.

—*Abraham Maslow*[4]

One of the most significant aspects of the new consciousness-based approach to healing is the systematic support of transformation. No longer just an accident of extreme circumstances, radical renewal of soul and body is seen as an accessible human potential, waiting to be activated. Through multi-dimensional, psycho-dynamic methods that penetrate the layers of culturalization, personal myth, and constricted belief systems that preclude successfully connecting with the greater Whole, transformation becomes the seed that grows new health. Spiritual harmony is now a legitimate therapeutic objective. The introspective psycho-technologies of meditation, visualization, invocation, and affirmations are recognized as viable healing tools.

THE NEW DOCTORS

If you are embarrassed by the word "spirit," think of spirit as the subtlest form of matter. But if you are not embarrassed by the word "spirit," then you can think of matter as the densest form of spirit.

—*Sri Aurobindo Ghose*

Some very significant, reliable results are being obtained by professionals approaching the problems of stress and disease with a holistic/spiritual perspective. This new breed of medical artist is not reluctant to acknowledge and work with the non-logical, emotional, subtle, and mysterious human soul. Progressive and innovative doctors are opening a rich new dimension in which healing can take place. Some of the influential forerunners in the new "empowerment medicine" include:

ELMER & ALYCE GREEN. The Greens founded the Voluntary Controls Program at the Menninger Foundation (Topeka). Influenced by the writings of Sri Aurobindo, they conducted the first controlled studies of yogic autonomic self-regulation in the United States (with Swami Rama, 1970). They established protocols in biofeedback that have led to its recognition as the treatment of choice for migraine headaches, Ryanaud's disease, hypertension, and other nervous system disorders. The Greens have made invaluable contributions in establishing such humanistic parameters as creativity, environment, relationship, and transpersonal factors as recognizable medical variables. By conducting cross-cultural studies, such as comparisons between Native American and East Indian beliefs, they have distilled important universal principles that have stood the test of time and vindicate the notion of a spiritual basis for healing. Among these are the unity of all life; man's connection to the Universe; the existence and role in healing of non-physical energies in living organisms; and the primary role of consciousness, volition and mental powers.

DR. RUDOLPH BALLENTINE and staff at the Himalayan Institute (Honesdale, Penn.). One of the first of its kind, this rural residential healing center has successfully combined the best of modern Western bio-technology, such as blood analysis and biofeedback, with ancient East Indian healing methods including yoga, meditation, and ayurvedic herbology to create a truly integrated whole-person therapeutic environment. The Himalayan Institute was founded by Swami Rama, and promotes a philosophy of health firmly based on inner spiritual growth and self-realization. Natural vegetarian diet, personal counseling, and the study of inspirational and metaphysical literature are important aspects of the program.

KENNETH PELLETIER, PH.D. Author of the classic, *Mind as Healer, Mind as Slayer,* and many other leading edge books on holistic health, Ken Pelletier has combined an open mind, careful research and the persuasive power of personal example, and succeeded in placing consciousness, stress management, self-care, and prevention on the new agenda of medicine in the eighties. He is an assistant clinical professor at the University of California School of Medicine and an active contributor to many health-oriented publications. His latest works deal with longevity and health in the workplace.

DOLORES KRIEGER, PH.D., R.N. A professor of nursing with extensive knowledge of holistic and cross-cultural methods,

Dr. Krieger also had a lifetime of training in spiritual healing with Theosophist Dora Kunz. She has taught Therapeutic Touch (an "energy-based" diagnostic and treatment modality) to some 10,000 student-healers at New York University medical school and other centers nationwide. She is also the founder of the Nurse-Healers Association, and author of *Foundations for Holistic Health Nursing Practices: The Renaissance Nurse.* Because of her rigorous clinical research and controlled studies, Dr. Kriegar has become a major influence in the shift towards recognition of non-physical factors and spiritual methods within the medical establishment.

LAWRENCE LESHAN. Author of *You Can Fight For Your Life,* and an early pioneer in the field of psycho-oncology (he began his research in the 1950s), LeShan has spent years verifying the crucial role played by self-identity and the quest for personal meaning in the fight against cancer. Without explicit reference to religion or "spirit," he has led hundreds of patients to the discovery of a more authentic connection to their lives and world. LeShan's work is a powerful testament to the importance of love in the therapeutic relationship.

A NEW KIND OF MEDICINE MAN

Dr. Bernie Siegel, M.D., F.A.C.S. is something of a medical renegade. He's the Yale/New Haven Medical Center surgeon who's gone holistic/spiritual. In his proximity, dying people start to laugh, nurses applaud, and doctors often scowl in disapproval. He plays music in the operating rooms and talks to an invisible guide named George. By his own description, he's "a little bit crazy."

An established resident surgeon, Dr. Siegel radically altered the focus of his practice (and risked his reputation) after discovering holistic and spiritual principles in healing. Founder of Exceptional Cancer Patients (ECAP),[5] Dr. Siegel has become a major spokesperson in the movement to humanize the medical profession and bring spiritual values to the hospital setting. His book is called *Love, Medicine, and Miracles.*

Bernie Siegel's innovative branch of psycho-oncology (with acknowledgements to pioneers Carl and Stephanie Simonton, and Elisabeth Kubler-Ross) is unconventional to say the least. He comes on like a medical-comic-front-man for God. Very funny, but also extremely knowledgeable about human survival potentials.

Siegel's methods would have been considered unprofessional just a few years ago, but he has consistently demonstrated successes in extending survival rates as well as dramatically improving his patient's quality of life and peace of mind. His highly accurate assessments of patients' conditions and life-situations, often based primarily on their crayon drawings, attest to his skills as a psycho-diagnostician.

Bernie Siegel is a refreshing voice for holistic humanism in the sterile, impersonal halls of modern medicine. He has brought back the powerful elements of hope, will, and the human spirit to health care delivery. His treatments include generous doses of touch, tears, and humor. Says he, "If you want to get well, hug your doctor and call him by his first name!" His ECAP brochure talks of "the therapeutic role of love."

Dr. Siegel's premises are sensible enough, but have been largely ignored by mainstream medicine. For example, the notion that lifestyle can be a contributing factor in cancer as in many diseases, and that changes in lifestyle can therefore be healing. Even catastrophic disease can be "a blessing in disguise" if it is understood in the full context of one's life and used as an opportunity for real personal growth.

Attitudes, beliefs, self-image, emotions, and goals are likewise understood as factors relevant to the course of disease and recovery. Resentment, hate, despair, and depression, says Dr. Siegel, are "DIE" messages to your body, whereas love, hope, humor, peace, forgiveness, and prayer are "LIVE" messages.

Siegel's empathetic approach to the doctor/patient relationship painfully highlights the insufficiences of most. He sometimes strongly rebukes his colleagues for their aloofness. Author of "The Cancer Patient's Bill of Rights," he encourages his patients to talk back to their doctors! This feisty independence has been recognized as a personality factor associated with faster tumor shrinkage and higher remission rates.[6] Ironically, the doctor's nemesis, non-compliance, may very well be a good sign from the point of view of the patient's psychological survivability.

The Exceptional Cancer Patient reaches for information on how to live with the disease, how to improve one's self-image, ways to reduce stress and resolve conflict, and thus to direct vast resources of human energy toward the healing process.[7]

Dr. Siegel's approach utilizes stress management, psycho/emotional counseling, group work, biofeedback, music, meditation, visualization, art therapy, play, vitamins, and *"anything that works!"* A major therapeutic objective is the development of a positive attitude, the importance of which cannot be over-estimated. The patient's entire family is thoroughly involved in the treatment plan. ECAP itself consitutes a strong support community.

Since "terminal" is a subjective call, and often dangerous, due to its traumatic effects on the patient, Siegel has abandoned the term. He says there is no such thing as false hope; all hope is true. He is also fond of saying that there's no such thing as dying: *"You're either dead or you're alive!"*

A "terminal" prognosis is a matter of statistics, guesswork and opinion. What this final pronouncement *really* means is, "We don't know what else to do." There is more, however, that the patient can do, and people need to have the right to disagree with their doctor, about prognosis or treatment, without fear of being abandoned.

Irrespective of the time they may have remaining to them, ECAP patients learn to exercise control, explore new options, develop self-expression, and generally greatly improve the quality of their lives. In the process some become "too busy to be sick." Others find a happiness that may have eluded them for a lifetime, and then die in peace. All know that they were fortunate to find an ally like Bernie Siegel: a doctor who heals the soul.

QUOTES FROM A LECTURE--DR. BERNIE SIEGEL, M.D.

- Cancer is a sign to take a new road.
- I'm inviting people to learn how to live.
- Become a person, not a disease.
- Pain equals change.
- Little miracles are not hard to achieve.
- There's no such thing as false hope.
- Live as if you're going to die tomorrow: You'll have so much fun you won't be able to!
- Change the rest of your life, clear your conscience, and take Vitamin C!
- I don't tell people to stop smoking, I just tell them to love themselves.
- If nobody loves you, and you can't love yourself, you're in trouble.
- Your subconscious mind knows what's going on in your body. The central nervous system and the immune system are one.
- The mind leads the way, to illness or to health.
- *When* you get sick is not a coincidence.
- Coincidence is God's way of remaining anonymous.

May 10, 1984. Cheshire County Hospital, Keene, NH.

VI.

IN YOGA AS IN LIFE

Yoga is self-knowledge, self-mastery, self-transformation.

Yoga is an ancient, natural method of mind/body self-care and development. Its benefits are numerous, including improvements in muscle elasticity, posture, blood circulation, and respiration, to name just a few. It is effective as both a preventive and corrective health routine for all body systems, including glandular, nervous, respiratory and digestive.

Today, yoga is helping not only young seekers, but over-stressed business people, housewives, olympic athletes, and recovering addicts improve their health and their lives. Through careful and regular practice of the yoga poses and movements appropriate to one's condition and abilities, it is often possible to gain greater flexibility, improve poor sleep patterns, and correct many minor (and some major) systemic and structural disorders, all without drugs or negative side effects.

The therapeutic value of yoga and its sister-science, meditation, is now well documented and rapidly gaining acceptance by such main-stream institutions as the insurance, medical and business communities, as well as by many performing artists and world-class athletes. It is almost universally endorsed as a sensible, reliable, and benign health improvement and maintenance regime.

It has become a cliche to say that yoga is thousands of

years old, but it truly is the great-grandfather of all the modern body/mind therapies. Yogis in India and Tibet were practicing auto-regulation of their sympathetic nervous systems ages before Western science conceded the possibility with the development of biofeedback. Likewise, autogenic training, visualization, self-hypnosis, progressive muscle relaxation, respiratory therapy, and even some modern dance and sports training methods can all claim yoga as their spiritual ancestor. Both its longevity and its recent rapid spread in the West say much about its appeal as a personal health care system.

Actually there are many "yogas," suiting the great variety of temperaments and aptitudes of human beings. What we in the West commonly call Yoga is the branch known as Hatha Yoga: the path of self-development which utilizes the most obvious, and readily available vehicle, the physical body.

HATHA YOGA

In my eleven years of teaching yoga, I have concluded that it is potentially valuable to a great number of people from all walks of life. The ages of my students have ranged from twelve to eighty, with physical conditions equally as varied. I have seen alcoholics, hypertensives, and people with heart disease, asthma, arthritis, and sciatica all show noticeable, and sometimes dramatic, improvement in specific symptoms and general health. Many had turned to yoga only after unsuccessful experiences with bio-medicine, osteopathy, and various "physical fitness" routines. Others came for the general, non-therapeutic benefits offered by yoga and were pleasantly surprised to realize just how much it could positively affect all aspects of their lives. Relaxation, flexibility, improved posture, greater energy, concentration, strength, and weight control are some of the results reported. People constantly tell me how important the classes are to their well-being.

One of my students, a professional potter, suffered for years from chronic back, neck and shoulder tension. After several months of slow, daily hatha yoga sessions, she became pain free. The experience has changed her entire outlook on life. Yoga is now a primary part of her lifestyle, and she does it as much for the "energy high" as for pain prevention.

Another student, a 48 year-old middle-class housewife and mother of eight, has become, within a few years, one of the most limber and flexible people I have ever known. She is now teaching yoga to beginners.

Unlike calisthenics, yoga is done slowly—the slower the better. It is not a cardio-vascular activity, although it is complementary to the more aerobic forms of physical fitness. An increasing number of coaches and athletes are discovering how the gentle practice of yoga, and the resilience it creates, enhances performance and reduces injuries, even in the more rigorous contact sports. Yoga also improves performance and safety in racquet games, jogging, swimming, biking, and most other sports.

Although it is not designed primarily for muscle building, increased strength is also a common result of the practice of yoga, due to its direct effects on muscle tissue. Stretching, relaxing, and massaging the muscles, as yoga does, brings more nutrients and oxygen to the individual cells and facilitates efficient removal of metabolic waste products, such as purine, uric acid, etc. It is the local build-up of these toxins that cause muscles to ache, weaken, and atrophy.

Note that the heart itself is virtually all muscle. Yoga especially benefits the heart in unique ways, giving it passive stimulation through inversions, abdominal lifts and churns, and deep breathing exercises. No other modality offers the benefits of such inner organ self-massage.

Hatha Yoga is based on positions (Sanskrit: *Asana)* as opposed to exercises. Very often the poses are held without movement, facilitating a deep release of tension and a corresponding feeling of increased "energy" characteristic of many holistic body therapies.* Emphasis is placed on the quality of attention one gives to the inner experience as well

---

* Sanskirt: prana, shakti, kundelini;   Chinese: chi;   Japanese: ki.

as the procedure. Utilizing the natural laws of physics and gravity, leverage and dynamic tension, yoga offers a cooperative rather than forceful relationship to body parts and systems.

In yoga, mind is integrated with body activity in a deliberate way unknown in regular physical fitness routines. In calisthenics, for example, one could conceivably attain the same cardio-vascular training and muscle definition while conversing or watching TV during the workout. With yoga, if one is not silent and inner-directed, bringing the attention of the mind to the physical and energetic experience, much is missed and the benefits are minimized. No matter how rigorous or correct a pose, it is up to the mind to achieve stillness (Sanskrit: samadhi), the optimum condition for the flow of human psycho-bioenergetic life energies, and therefore, real healing. For this reason, it is not uncommon to observe yogis practicing with eyes closed. They are "listening" to the miraculous wisdom of their own life-force and its billion-year-old, trillion-celled self-regenerating genetic engine, the human body.

Yoga has also been introduced with great success in substance abuse rehabilitation, and in the prison setting.[3] My own work with alcoholics and youthful drug offenders confirms yoga's excellent reputation with such populations. It provides almost immediate demonstration of its validity to these out-of-shape beginners with noticeably short attention spans. (In other words, they feel good within the first hour!) Predictably, almost none will pursue the practice on their own, but within the context of a class of peers, yoga is both appealing and effective with people in institutional settings.

PAIN: THE YOGA APPROACH

One of the more unexpected and remarkable results of yoga practice is its modulating influence on one's experience of pain. Some body building methods aim at pain as a prerequisite for gain. Yoga offers a more positive way of understanding and relating to pain when it does arise.

Pain is actually a constellation of experiences, some of which we contribute to unwittingly through unskillful body/mind economy. Such mental factors as fear, aversion, negative imagination, and even egocentricity can exacerbate pain, and in many cases, cause an otherwise mild body sensation to feel painful. Pain is often a self-fulfilling prophecy.

This is well illustrated by the significant differences in childbirthing experiences between women who expect to go through "labor pains," and those who can anticipate and relate to that same experience as something like "birth rushes." Expectation and imagination are enormously powerful in determining quality of experience. We unwittingly fabricate much of our suffering by letting our unexamined mental habits run away with us.

The amorphous, mutable quality of "a pain" can become more apparent when examined with clear, focused attention, but our conditioning has made us habitually attempt to *avoid* pain at all cost. One cost is our understanding of the relativity of pain. This mental dimension to pain is now being explored, with excellent results, in the new drugless, autonomic/autogenic pain-control therapies, including meditation, biofeedback, hypnosis, and visualization techniques.[1]

I tell my yoga students to adopt a respectful, philosophical, and even playful attitude towards the "pain" of working at the edge of one's growth potential. The slow pace of yoga enables us to become aware, and *let go,* of that component of our physical discomfort which we have unconsciously added by manufacturing a collection of automatic, negative responses around the original sensation. In a meditative mind-set we can begin to discover that the "alarm response" to pain is a product of the higher, interpretive functions of the mind, which is in the habit of assigning meaning to our raw sensory data. It becomes possible to "uncouple" the cognitive, reactive mind from the sensory-receptor brain. When this happens, the afferent-efferent cycle is broken, self-agitation is reduced, and the "pain" is acknowledged, examined, and accepted as it *really* is: usually not nearly as bad as we *imagined.* Physically, this also has the result of subtracting the stress factors from the sum total of the "pain" experience. Through the power of careful attention we can discover pain's subjective qualities and quite naturally revise our relationship to it.

I've had some very practical opportunities to utilize yogic mind-control techniques with some of the common pains of life, including back aches, head aches, and heart aches! My dentist has been greatly intrigued by my calm acceptance of root-canal work without any anesthetic. I have learned to practice yoga when and where it is necessary.

Achieving such equanimity in pain control merely involves learning and practicing the various yogic techniques of breathing, relaxation, concentration, and other time-tested autonomic self-regulation methods. Yoga offers to anyone willing to make the commitment of time and discipline, nothing less than the transmutation of suffering into knowledge and understanding, and the transcendence of one's self-assumed limitations.

In hatha yoga this often means extending a pose to a point previously thought not possible, not by forcing the body into submission, but by slowly relaxing into the deeper stretch. It is an empowering and enlightening experience to overcome personal physical limits, *by relaxing past them.* This is felt when the outward force working on the body (either gravity or isolated muscle power) is met with interior surrender of the habitual tension surrounding the area being worked. In this way, many yoga poses are ingenious postural arrangements whereby one passive part of the body can be stretched or strengthened by another active part, in an inner, cooperative release.

In the broadest sense, yoga *is* self-healing. The list is long of common systemic disorders that can be eliminated or greatly alleviated through the correct and diligent practice of yoga over an extended period of time. This is because the changes that yoga induces in the body—muscle stretching, oxygenation, glandular stimulation, waste elimination—all give powerful positive support to the body's own regenerative and recuperative abilities.

There are, however, a few contra-indications for hatha yoga. These include: acute spinal dislocations, phlebitis, embolisms, neuro-vascular disorders, and osteoporosis. People with migraines, glaucoma, and coronary problems should avoid the inversions. Pregnant women should have medical consultation and expert supervision. Those with hypertension can approach yoga with hope, for it calms the cardio-vascular and nervous systems, but caution would be in order when doing inversions and deep breathing. Have your doctor monitor your progress.

Arthritis sufferers should do as much range-of-motion exercises as possible, in spite of the pain. The disease is unique in that working *against* the pain is necessary. The joints are like rusty hinges. Movement breaks calcification and stimulates the production of synovial fluid at the wearing surfaces (*Use 'em or lose 'em!*) Passive traction and range-of-motion also helps the joints. The way to handle the pain, and gauge how much to take is learning to *relax into* it. Resistant muscles, restricted breathing, and grimacing are all indicators that you are proceeding too quickly. Ease up on the pose until you can relax. In yoga, the measure of your gain is not how hard you can push (masculine, Western, left brain, controlling), but how easily and thoroughly you can surrender (feminine, Eastern, right brain, cooperating).

It wasn't until I sustained a serious back injury that I came to know the therapeutic powers of yoga first hand. A congenital anomaly in my spine, agravated by several childhood mishaps and a high school football injury, had led to a degenerating disk and a forward subluxation of the fifth lumbar vertebrae.

One morning when I was in my mid-twenties I woke up totally immobilized by shooting pains in my lower back. I literally crawled for help, for my spine could not support my own weight. The pain was so sharp it took my breath away. My old childhood injury had come back with a vengeance. It would challenge all my resources to recover my strength and mobility.

Several weeks of pain would pass before I would be able to lead any semblance of a normal life. I moved about with a cane like an old man. Luckily I knew about the benefits of chiropractic. If I hadn't I might have complied with a hospital physician's advice to have spinal surgery, with no guarantee of improvement. I opted for the less radical and invasive approach of structural self-rehabilitation, and, to borrow a phrase, that has made all the difference.

Basically, chiropractic is the manual re-alignment of displaced spinal vertebrae. When the misalignment is causing pressure on a nerve, such as the sciatic, a chiropractic "adjustment" can bring dramatic relief. When I first experienced this kind of help, I established a great respect for this practical, manual healing art. I was lucky to have found my way to the office of a chiropractor who had healing in his hands, and he taught me much about my body's own repairability, and set the stage for my lifelong involvement with yoga.

Yoga and chiropractic have much in common, particularly, an understanding of the special significance of the spine to overall health. Both are natural, low-risk body manipulations which align the spine, relieve nerve pressure, counteract chronic muscle tension, and therefore induce improved circulation and organ function. The importance of posture, exercise and relaxation are also common denominators relating yoga and chiropractic.

Of course one key difference between chiropractic and yoga is that the latter is done alone. Hatha yoga utilizes poses, breathing exercises, concentration, and relaxation techniques as tools that greatly extend the individual's ability to fix and fine-tune his or her system. In many ways, yoga is auto-chiropractic. I discovered many of the poses by pursuing my body's own craving for position-specific relief.

The outcome of my experience with a severe spinal injury was complete recovery and an enormous sense of gratitude for having been exposed to the principles of natural, therapeutic bodywork. It was my great fortune to have my disability lead me to something resembling that fountain of youth which everyone's been looking for! Today my love for yoga translates into disease prevention and personal longevity training. I look at it as a kind of free health insurance.

YOGA AS "PERSON BUILDING"

Yoga not only feels good, but it makes organic sense to the body's genetic memory of itself. It is not something we "get" from a teacher, so much as a discovery of the natural, organic wisdom already residing deep within, waiting to be heard. Proof of this inherent naturalness is the fact that children often spontaneously perform yoga poses without ever being introduced to the practice. Even animals "do yoga," and many of the positions are named after wild creatures, illustrating its primal relationship to nature. Observe, or better yet, imitate, the way a dog bows and stretches when it first arises from sleep and you will get an intuitive understanding of the yoga pose called "The Downward-Facing Dog."

Emphasizing this inherent "rightness" of yoga in my classes, I encourage newcomers and experienced students alike to bypass the self-judging mind and consult their intuition and body-sense, rather than authorities and books, about the validity of an exercise for them. Yoga is a constant personal internal dialogue with this deeper level of organic knowledge, one which, if carefully cultivated, enables us to virtually *take lessons from within.* Yoga is a way of listening. It's only after some regularity and internalization of the practice that one recognizes that talking about the benefits, powers, and joys of yoga is really talking about the benefits, powers, and joys of oneself! It's a phenomenal realization, one that I particularly enjoy seeing my students go through. Ultimately, and in every sense, yoga is nothing else but You.

As opposed to just "body building," yoga is really "person building." It is not merely positions or exercises. Yoga is a way of being, in one's body and in the Universe. Beyond its therapeutic and rehabilitative applications, the greatest benefits of yoga are in the realm of developing positive, human potential. Reflecting its spiritual roots as an ancient practice of liberation and self-realization (Sanskrit: *nirvana*), yoga accelerates the personal evolution of the committed practitioner. The "side effects" of this quest go far beyond mere alleviation of illness to improvements in self esteem, learning skills, creativity, and intuition.

The potential transformation which yoga offers is multi-dimensional. Besides the numerous physiological benefits mentioned above, hatha yoga facilitates the generation and circulation of the etheric life-energy/force (Sanskrit: *prana*) in the whole human body, and particularly in the seven energy centers of the spine.

"*Ha*" means sun and "*tha*" means moon, reflecting the dynamic quality of yoga and its emphasis on *balance.* Again, the implications go well beyond the first, physical stage, for a truly balanced person is one who is at peace. Balance is manifested in life as poise, equanimity, and a certain skill in negotiating life's challenges. A basic premise in the yogic and meditative traditions is that such refined human qualities are not merely appointments of fate, but are predictable psycho-spiritual manifestations of conscientious work on one's self (Sanskrit: *Sadhana*).

"Yoga" means union (as in "yoke"). Ultimately it points beyond such dualistic distinctions as body and mind, energy and matter, creation and creator, subject and object. It promotes the integration of all human faculties and capacities. Importantly, union in the yogic sense also connotes union with the Ultimate: The transcendent spiritual wisdom and freedom wherein one's deepest/highest nature and that of the Universe are realized as One. Regardless of the reasons people have for "taking yoga," whatever physical benefits it may produce are secondary and incidental to this potential for spiritual growth and self-realization.

Although our discussion is ostensibly about bodily health,

one should realize that this is actually a co-effect of yoga. In more complete transformations related to the long-term practice of yoga, there may be para-psychological and trans-personal results as well. These include conscious dreaming, precognition, telepathy, "deja vu" and serendipitous experiences ("cosmic coincidences"), out-of-body experiences, and other non-ordinary states of awareness and "knowing." Until quite recently, these phenomena have been dismissed as too aberrant or "soft" for science to study seriously. But yoga itself is a science (a "psycho-technology") in every sense of the word: a verifiable relationship between cause (the practice) and its effects on health and human performance. What one clinical investigator may see as "para-normal," a practitioner knows to be lawful. We are only now coming to understand, through the studies of humanistic and transpersonal psychology, attitudinal healing, and the human potential movement, just how much we've underestimated the miraculous powers of human self-improvement. These "soft" sciences are now pointing the way beyond the physical limitations of bio-medicine.

VII.

CORE RELAXATION

Let go of everything you can think of.   —*a meditation master*

Core relaxation is the deepest relaxation possible. It involves interior as well as exterior muscle release, and is felt down to the cellular level, as opposed to only in large muscle groups. As you will see, it combines several effective relaxation/auto-regulation techniques.

This constellation of strategies includes postural balance, neuro-motor quieting, passive breath techniques, and energy awareness. Combined, they make up a total psycho-physiological experience, and tend to bring about full integration of body, mind, and energy.

Core relaxation is the art of throwing your metabolism into neutral and coasting on its miraculous natural momentum. It is basic to the meditative therapies and is essential in achieving the "theta" brain wave pattern associated with optimal training in biofeedback, visualization, hypnosis, and other psychodynamic modalities. It also tends to greatly increase one's proprioceptive and somasthetic awareness of, and control over, internal body functions. In this way, our bodies can speak to us, daily reporting on potential problems and guiding us to accurate, preventative choices.

Physiologically, core relaxation is an optimal strategy for pain management, eyesight improvement, natural birthing, biofeedback training, developing balance, good sleep, and even easier dying. Practicing it tends to place one in harmony with the Universe (Chinese: *Tao*).

Because our minds are almost always processing thoughts, memories, anxieties, and a million other mind pictures per second, much of our psycho-neurologically sensitive systems and organs rarely rest, as biofeedback monitoring readily demonstrates. This chronic background agitation takes an enormous toll in human nervous energy, with or without our being aware of it. With core relaxation techniques, we can place the entire organism on idle, quieting all dimensions of our being, material and subtle, systemic to cellular, neuro-electric to biomagnetic, and on the atomic level as well.

PREPARTORY STRETCHING

As with many inner-directed techniques, it is easiest to arrive at stillness by beginning with a few good stretches. Get all your impulses to move "out of your system" before attempting to do deep relaxation. Isometric flexing of the muscles will help discharge residual tension, and slow deep breathing can set the necessary tone for the stillness to follow. Take a seated position, with the spine erect, but not uptight. You should have the feeling of settling down, through the spine, into your seat.

BALANCE AND CENTERING

Our "sense of balance" is a faculty that can be enlisted to great advantage on the way to deep states of relaxation and healing. Like breathing, it operates close to the interface between mind and body and reveals their intimate dialog. If you are seeking equanimity and composure of *mind*, a good strategy is to develop balance of *body*. Balance means literally and metaphorically, *where are you coming from?* If you can learn to remain "centered" in yourself, chances are you will be better equipped to handle the vicissitudes of life. Balance is an antidote to stress-overload.

Begin by tuning in to your three axes of position: front-to-back, side-to-side, and up-and-down. Slowly and carefully bring your awareness to the midpoints of each of these three axes within you, and to the center where they all intersect; i.e., your center of gravity. This point, as is well known in the oriental martial arts, lies at the level of the solar plexus (Japanese: *hara*) and coincides with the origin of the breath. Many eastern traditions take this location to be the seat of the soul. Use it to bring your awareness to the "center" within.

As described in the section on breathing, use passive breathing to locate the stillpoint between breath-motions. Practice coming to rest within this moment of complete passivity, while at the same time re-creating the other stages of core relaxation: deep muscle release, balance, and centering. All of these inner actions should occur at once (and repeatedly), engendering a full, unifying experience of deep core relaxation. Allow it to wash over and through you in waves.

PROGRESSIVE DEEP RELEASE

Progressive Muscle Relaxation (PMR) has been described in detail in the section on stress reduction. Basically, it is a systematic relinquishing of muscle tension, usually done in cooperation with the downward pull of gravity, starting with the major limbs and working into finer levels of neuro-muscular release.

Deeper levels of PMR are achieved by becoming aware of and deliberately relaxing specific internal body parts which are not usually sensed or controlled. Each cycle of scanning and releasing brings the body into a more dormant, but also more sensitive state. While at this level, the sensations feel more like energy release than mechanical adjustment. It is suggested that the progression then be from the bottom up, as if you can sense a fountain of energy originating at the base of the spine.*

---

* Those familiar with the Eastern chakra-yoga system will recognize its influence in this integration with the Western psycho-biological model.

GENITAL & RECTAL MUSCLES. One good indicator for core relaxation is the degree of release attainable deep within the pelvic region. The action of the genital and rectal muscles are closely linked and can be readily relaxed once they can be sufficiently sensed under voluntary control. This may take some practice.

Begin by using the "Kegel" exercise: tighten the area as if restricting urination. Then open up all the involved muscles as if emptying yourself completely. (Obviously, the bladder and bowels must be voided beforehand.) If practiced regularly, this exercise will strengthen the sphincter muscles, thus preventing hemorrhoids. It also has the added benefit of toning up the sex glands and increasing sensitivity and control in this area. Note that throughout these discussions of auto-regulatory techniques and inner awareness, the concept of "emptying" applies psycho-metaphorically as well as physically.

Due to cultural conditioning, many people have a negative or repressive relationship with their own sexual and eliminative functions. Although this is usually unconscious, the subsequent tension and relative reduction of feeling in the pelvic region is commonplace, often reflected in rigidity, various sexual dysfunctions, constipation, and even cancer. The discovery of correlations of such physical problems with childhood stress, such as traumatic toilet training experiences, or severe parental and religious sanctions against sexual self-pleasure, illustrates the power of indoctrinated fear in determining musculature, circulation, organ function and overall health.*

In yoga psychology, those that tend to deny and repress their natural sexuality, as well as those that are obsessed with it (most of us!) are said to be "stuck" in the second chakra (energy center). It helps to relate to one's sexual energy as but one form of the universal force which animates us, and all life,

---

* Credit for the introduction of these ideas to the West belongs to pioneer body therapist Wilhelm Reich, who was severely persecuted in the 1950's for advocating a liberating, psycho-sexual approach to disease, particularly cancer. His books were burned, and Reich died in prison for his conviction that sex is healthy.[1]

on the way to total consciousness. The optimal strategy for growth here is to acknowledge and accept yourself as a sexual being, while at the same time opening to "higher" levels. While physically relaxing the rectal and genital muscles, simultaneously allow your attention to flow up and out towards the next level, the abdominal region.

ABDOMEN & DIAPHRAGM. This area is one of the most reactive to stress, and vital to deep inner calm. It is impossible to relax any further than what the belly and breath will allow. Learning how to release tension from this area can create profound healing changes throughout the system.

To gain a good sense of awareness and control, tighten the abdominal muscles first, and then loosen them thoroughly, cooperating with the sensation of softness which spreads over and through the area. This "quieting reflex" will reach the diaphragm muscle itself when you can feel as if you are surrendering your exhalations completely, as in Passive Breath Awareness (PBA). Practice letting the outbreath fall away, as far as possible, without effort, and allow the resulting open stillness to spread from within.

The abdominal area is very sensitive to one's social/emotional situations. This is the physical focus of our responses to competition, manipulation, politics, status, money, property, fame, etc. It is no wonder that the business world is the spawning ground for ulcers, given the relationship between stress and digestion.

Psychologically, the life of the gut is marked by a dualistic view of the world: me versus them. It is the source of boundary-defining, appropriate to the level of evolution of the hunter and the organs of digestion, both of which need to distinguish "self" from other in order to function properly. Halfway between our animal and God natures, the human ego has the potential for being the instrument of cooperation and community. To best negotiate this realm, it is necessary to learn the distinction between self-assertiveness, an important social skill, and its distorted extreme form, domination. When we deliberately and imaginatively invoke and nurture feelings of trust, defenses dissolve, and relaxation (especially of the abdominal and lower back muscles) easily follows.

The primal element in chakra symbolism for this area is fire ("solar" plexus), appropriate when we realize that heat-generating aerobic digestion occurs here. Due to the inherent prioritizing of biological functions in our systems during survival situations, stress often causes a postponement of digestion in favor of immediate self-defense mechanisms. Therefore, under emergency conditions, blood and body temperature move away from the hollow organs, outward towards the muscular periphery. Hence, stress equals poor digestion and "low fire" (energy)—one good reason to abstain from eating when upset. Inner relaxation techniques reverse this syndrome, making the system more efficient, releasing energy. (We can be purified in the fire, without burning out!)

HEART. As indicated in the autogenic exercise instructions, the heart is a muscle that is at last partially responsive to self-programming and imagery. One useful technique is to simply keep one's focus on the heart beating in the chest, and imagine that it feels as if it is slowing down. It soon does follow the mental expectation, a classic autogenic response. Imagine a feeling of increased circulation throughout the chest cavity. In a short time, what you feel will no longer be a figment of your imagination. Even though such changes originate in the mind, their metabolic effects are verifiable through biofeedback. There's no such thing as "just your imagination": Every psychological event is reflected in the body.

Holistic therapists now recognize the importance of the symbolic/reflective (i.e. psycho-somatic) dynamic between body and mind, as when grieving people actually *feel* their heart ache. Conversely, invoking the positive feelings commonly associated with this vital organ seems to have a calming effect: Picture before you someone you love unconditionally, and feel as if your heart is "opening." Emotions turn out to be one of the keys to organ activity and health.

Psychologically, the heart represents the first level at

which we have the opportunity to transcend the personal ego. The emotional "qualities" of the heart have to do with love, compassion, and altruism. Appropriately, the element associated with the chest area is air, the element that most clearly demonstrates the inside-out nature of our interdependence with the world.

You can open and develop the heart center by meditatively cultivating unconditional love for someone you know, and then gradually expanding the feeling by adding more people in widening circles of compassion. Practice this until you can imagine all beings in your heart (including your enemies!). It's also useful to picture a radiant, healing light flowing from the center of your chest, especially during exhalation. Now let a color which looks and feels healing spontaneously suggest itself. Envision more of this colored energy pouring into your heart with every inhalation, and out with every exhalation. Breathing should be slow and easy.

EPIGLOTTIS & LARYNX. Another sensitive area that can act as a key to the sympathetic nervous system includes the epiglottis (the valve that prevents us from breathing our food), and the "voice box" (larynx). This region is best relaxed by allowing the jaw to drop and gently sighing out the sound "ahh." Feel softness and warmth spread from the throat area throughout the neck and shoulders. Make sure the head is balanced so that all the neck and shoulder muscles can be permitted to relax. This is also the location of the thyroid gland, a master regulator and coordinator of glandular functions. You can visualize healing colors moving in and through the thyroid and positively affecting the entire endocrine system.

Holistic therapists have recognized that the throat and jaw are often the site of unexpressed, negative feelings, particularly of anger. People literally lock their jaws when not able to speak their minds, becoming at risk for bruxism, temporo-mandibular joint syndrome (TMJ), torticollis, and possibly thyroid dysfunctions, due to local oxygen deficiency and chronic structural distortion. Facial and upper body massage is recommended in such cases. In a holistic program, enhancing communication skills and greater self-esteem would be therapeutic goals. Improvements in speech patterns and voice quality would be expected indicators of positive response, as would be more authentic self-expression and creativity.

Also beneficial to the throat region is the use of chanting, and sonic intoning. One Tibetan practice entails sounding the deepest note possible immediately upon arising in the morning, when the vocal cords are most relaxed. The feeling of "clearing" which this creates in the thoracic cavity is remarkable. Try softly and smoothly sounding out the single syllable "OM" nonstop for fifteen minutes, and you will experience the effects of what the shamans call "sonic driving." I have had the good fortune of participating in all-night chanting ceremonies in both the Native American and East Indian traditions. The sense of spiritual renewal, energy, peace and understanding that follow such practices cannot be described.

EYES. Eye movement, like many of the sensitive automatic mechanisms in the body, responds readily to the use of imagination in de-stressing procedures. Visualization is especially effective at this level. The eyes tend to activate or relax according to mental events almost as readily as to light stimulation. Rapid Eye Movement (REM) during sleep is a good example of this phenomenon: All the eye adjustments are appropriate to the mind-events in dreams—a perfect illustration of mind/body "mirroring." This indicates some of the potentials of image-based healing.

If you close your eyes, but "picture" something like a printed page before you, the ciliary muscles will constrict the iris and shape the lens as if appropriately responding to the light-stimulation of the imagined scene. In the case of core relaxation, precisely the opposite is desired: All the minute muscles and nerves within and about the eyes are put at absolute rest. This is done, in effect, by *picturing nothing!*

George Leonard calls this "soft eyes." There is no trying to see anything. When this happens, a distinct physical sensation, a "felt shift" is experienced.

Here is a simple progressive eye relaxation and healing procedure: Close your eyes and imagine viewing a tree in the distance. Now imagine looking, not at anything in particular, but at the whole landscape in general, with a very soft, unfocused gaze. Then, instead of thinking of yourself as "looking," just allow the "seen" to come in, becoming purely visually receptive. Finally, allow your imaginary sky to grow progressively darker, diffusing into night. This will automatically dilate the pupils and relax the eyes.

You can take this response one step further by imagining the sockets and optic nerves behind the eyes also feeling the relaxation. Although there are no actual muscles here, you can induce an unmistakable soothing sensation, even into the brain itself. Just imagine how it would feel to relax your brain, and you will soon feel it. Remember to breathe freely. This technique works well for headache relief.

In the esoteric traditions, the "Third Eye" (between the eyebrows) is felt to be the seat of the "sixth sense": intuition, telepathy, and the perception of transpersonal phenomena. Here is a typical visualization to develop this level:

With eyes closed, gaze softly at the inside of the forehead center, with a non-analytical gaze, as into a thick fog at night. Spend a few moments resting the eyes in this soft darkness. Then imagine a dawning light, followed by a golden sunrise on a horizon. Feel its healing light-energy penetrate your inner eye and spread throughout your brain. Become transparent to the brilliance, allowing it to dispel every trace of darkness within you. "Become" the Light.

Following the procedure outlined above will enable you to sense your inner metabolism in ways not accessible in everyday, active life. The entire circulatory system, for example, can be sensed as surging blood throughout your body. The interpenetrating network of nerves can also be felt: calm, yet charged with life energies. These energies can be mobilized by the mind to any local area in need of healing. You can use simple visualization to "picture" (and feel) improvement happening instantly. Even though these ideas will initially be manufactured concepts, you can soon fully enter the actual embodied experience to which they refer. You really can become the source of your own infinite power, but the more you tap, the more important it becomes to practice centering and relaxation techniques.

The consummation of the core relaxation process is realized when you can feel perfectly balanced in mind and body, and are no longer *doing* anything, on any level. You are simply *being*, with open awareness, pure alert receptivity permeated with deep peace. In fact, your sense of separateness may completely disappear.

In India, yogis have developed a meditative method of auto-sensory-deprivation, called "pratyahara." Essentially, it's a systematic voluntary shutting down of all sensory input, leaving awareness undisturbed and undefined, in its inherent condition of pure, free ("original") potential receptivity. Significantly, thought itself is dealt with as a kind of sense, which can be shut down. Then consciousness comes closer to self-knowledge (Tibetan: *Bodhi:* "enlightened mind").

In the technological West, sensory deprivation is achieved with devices such as isolation tanks, masking feedback, and even certain types of drugs. To a person used to identifying with the objects of sense, i.e., the exterior world, sensory deprivaton can be terrifying. To a transpersonally-oriented meditator, it is a rather blissful experience of dwelling in a greatly heightened/expanded state.

The longer one remains in such a suspended state, and the more frequently it is entered, the more efficiently the body's own powerful self-healing abilities can function. The efficiency of self-repair in conscious, meditative deep relaxation is far greater than what sleep alone allows.

In summary, core relaxation entails a release of the energy bound up in chronic physical and mental tension, releasing it from throughout the system, even well into the body's central nerve-core, the spinal column. The complete sequence, including preparatory relaxation, moves from the top down, the outside in, and finally from the bottom up, as the feeling of deep relaxation permeates your entire being on progressively finer levels of awareness. The approach is one of the opposite to effort. That is, we surrender, release, and otherwise completely relinquish our usual grip on ourselves, with the paradoxical result of gaining significantly more energy with which to positively enhance our lives.

VIII.

THE PICTURE OF HEALTH

. . . all intentional transformation starts with the idea of change. To that idea we add our emotion, and finally, the "vital energy" is reflexively activated. It begins to modify and regenerate the cellular structure of the body. —*Sri Aurobindo*

The more we investigate, the more certain it seems that the most important "medium" of the mind is pictures. Although we usually assume that the mind's content is simply made up of thoughts, a careful look reveals that most of these interior events—thoughts, memories, plans, reflections, all the mental conversations we have with ourselves—are *seen* graphically (more accurately, holographically) by consciousness. The mind is both the projector of all this visual material, and the witness to it. Many psychologists, as well as philosophers, believe that a visual idea precedes every human activity, conscious or otherwise. Envisioning may well be a primary determinant of our definition of reality. It certainly has a bearing on our health.

Presently there is much excitement being generated within the brain/mind scientific community over the discovery of the synergetic/therapeutic effects of relaxation and visualization. The dynamic coupling of these two modalities has ramificatons in fields of learning, creativity, and optimal performance. Many world class athletes now use mental-imaging techniques, known as Visual Motor Behavioral Rehearsal. The approach has resulted in measurable improvement in a wide range of sports that demand high concentration and neuro-motor coordination.[1]

But by far the most promising possibilities for visualization are in the area of self-induced healing. Visualization has become standard in stress reduction classes, and is rapidly establishing its place among the viable new approaches to hypertension, gastric disorders, migraine, diabetes, arthritis, cancer, and even broken bones. Children with hemophilia have been taught how to go into light trance and stop bleeding by "seeing" their blood coagulate, and cancer patients are now using visualization to reduce the negative side effects of chemotherapy and radiation treatments, including pain, nausea, and even hair loss. The successful use of hypnosis and visualization for spontaneous wart removal is a legendary enigma in medical circles.

The study of the positive influence of imagery on the immune system is the providence of the fledgling science with the composite name of psychoneuroimmunology. For the first time, science is beginning to map the mysterious territory between the mind and brain, and it is finding direct applications in healing. Healing imagery video tapes are now available.[2]

Medical imagery researchers Jeanne Achterberg and Frank Lawliss have consistantly found higher remission rates and more successful recovery among cancer patients who can learn to clearly visualize their ailment, treatment, and improvement.[3] They were able to identify both high prognostic indicators and high recovery predictors in cancer patient's own imagery and drawings. These include the colors, vividness, activity, and strength of the symbols used, as well as the degree of emotional investment in the images.

"Picturing" turns out to be one of the keys to the door between the automatic functioning, repair, and defense of the cells, and the full awareness of the organism—and it often makes the difference in terms of survival. Here is an account by Elmer and Alyce Green of what one patient was able to do with interior "viewing" under hypnosis:

One day it occurred to Dr. H. that this particular patient would be a good one with whom to try blood-flow control through hypnosis. Because of urinary complications, a catheter had been installed to relieve pressure in the bladder, and the blood-and-urine mixture in the transparent catheter tube gave an immediate indication of the amount of hemorrhaging in the cancerous area. While in deep trance, the patient was told that a control center in the middle of the brain regulated all the blood vessels of the body. Could he find it? After a short time he said yes. When asked what it looked like he described something like a boiler room full of pipes, or perhaps the inside of a submarine. There were valves, switches, and control levers for regulating pipes of all sizes.

Dr. H. told the patient that one of the pipes controlled blood flow in the cancer on the bladder and that if he could locate that pipe and its control valve, it would be beneficial to turn it off. Soon the man reported that he had found the valve and pipe—it was labeled—and after a few seconds he said that he had turned it off. The two doctors were very much impressed when in a short time there was a sharp line of demarcation between clear urine and the previous mixture of urine and blood coming down the catheter tube.

The bleeding was almost entirely stopped within a week, and the patient's appetite returned. After another week the patient said that he wanted to go home (he was admitted as a terminal case). He said that the growth on the bladder, which had been described as being about the size of a grapefruit, was shrinking and now was only about the size of an orange. Since his health continuously improved, his stays at home became longer. Eventually he reported to the hospital only once a month.[2]

A wide variety of possible "visualizations" for self-healing are available through books, tapes, and trained facilitators and counselors. Two main types are guided imagery and intuitive visualization. In the former, healing scenarios and symbols are suggested by the facilitator, or the practitioner "programs" an agreed-upon self-healing image. This works well with groups as well as individuals. Intuitive visualization is more self-reliant and subjective, but requires some training in concentration and the important principles of self-programing. A combination of the two approaches within one session can be particularly fruitful: That is, after creating the visual setting and the necessary mood and receptivity through narration, the patient calls up her own imagery as a personal, authoritative source of vital information from the subconscious. This can be used in a kind of intuitive auto-diagnosis. *Ask your body what it needs, then look and listen.*

For effective medical imagery, it is important that the scene imagined be "egosyntonic": consistant with the true character, beliefs, desires, and values of the patient. Bernie Siegel tells of one patient who walked out of his doctor's office when offered a drug designed to *kill* his cancer. The man was a Quaker and completely committed to pacifism. The drawings of the imagery he decided to use in therapy showed his white blood cells carefully, almost respectfully, carrying out the sick cancer cells one at at time! The man recovered.

Mind pictures for healing can be symbolic, but they should be anatomically consistant. It's better, for instance, to picture the macrophage cells enveloping the cancer cells (which they do), as opposed to injecting them with poison (which they do not). The scenario should have a positive outcome. Additionally, it should be experienced as within the body, and have kinesthetic and sensory qualities (feelings as opposed to just thought/pictures). One method is so deliberate as to co-ordinate four phases of visualized imagery (scene setting, preparation, action, and result) with the four phases of the breath: inbreath, upper interlude, outbreath, lower interlude.[3] Finally, to be successful, healing visualization must be done repeatedly, with commitment and will.

A visualization session typically includes physical relaxation exercises, such as Autogenics and/or PMR, a mental progression into deep, internal relaxation (using gradual-induction imagery such as descending escalators, etc.), the mental creation of a vivid multi-sensory setting in a peaceful, calming environment, and finally the healing phase itself, which consists of healing activities, images, symbols, messages, etc., either given or elicited. Certain types of consciously created music are very conducive to visualization. The results often include conflict resolution, release of "blockages" and a sense of increased energy. This inner release/transformation (also known as a "felt shift") is the essential *raison d'etre* and power of holistic visualization techniques, and often leads to physical improvement.

HEALING IMAGES

Here are some typical healing images for specific health problems. Please note that they are intended to augment, not replace other sound methods of cure. Their effects may be subtle, dramatic, or simply nonexistent, depending upon a host of individual variables. Remember that visualization should follow deep relaxation to be most effective.

These instructions will sound disturbingly simplistic to a good medical skeptic. The wise will try them and judge for themselves. Someday it will be understood that it is no more difficult to communicate with the organs of the body than it was to grow them. We have only just discovered that the medium of communication is visual/emotive.

- Infection: Picture a body part that is healthy; imagine that healthy feeling spreading to the infected area. Picture the millions of antibodies in your blood swiftly and efficiently immobilizing and disposing of foreign micro-organisms.
- Headache: Specifically locate the pain. Assess its size, shape, and color, if any. Then as you exhale, imagine the pain going out through the nearest orifice. Repeat as needed.
- Cold, or Stuffy Sinuses: Imagine the tubes leading from your sinuses to your nose opening up and the fluid draining out like a sink unclogging. Picture the channels of

your lymph system dilating. (Postural drainage works well too: You can visualize while horizontal or inverted.)

● Cuts, or Broken Bones: Imagine healthy, new cells filling in the gaps like bricks being laid by a mason. Picture tendrils, branches, and then bridges of new tissue spanning the wound and filling it in. Do infection-prevention visualizations.

● Angina or Overly Fast Heartbeat: Visualize yourself on a beautiful, calm, deserted beach, getting healed by the sun, air, and ocean. Imagine the feeling of your heart beating slowly and easily. Say to yourself that's how it feels. Feel supported by the earth and universe.

● Sore Throat. Imagine the back of your throat becoming pink, slightly moist and more comfortable. Summon fresh blood and immune factors to the area. Imagine sighing out the soothing sound "aahhh."

● Skin Rash: Picture your skin becoming smooth, soft, and normal in color. Send energy to the surface of your body. Imagine you can sense the thousands of pores in your skin opening and breathing. Use cooling images.

● Lower Back Pain: Lie down and imagine your lower spine becoming heavier, your muscles flattening and lengthening. Envision knots unwinding. See the spaces between your vertebrae open.

● Asthma. Visualize the millions of alveoli in your lungs relaxing and dilating. Imagine the air inside you as cool and light.

Once you get the gist of how this kind of corrective visualization works, it's useful to custom-make your own images. In general, the idea is to picture and otherwise imagine sensing how improvement in the area in question would look and feel. For weak organs, visualize energy. For tension, imagine softness; for heat, cold, etc. Use color in your images.

When working with pain, carefully analyze the pain in order to get a clear "picture" of its particular characteristics, e.g.: like a sharp knife, a knotted rope, a hot poker. Then devise exactly the visual image that would positively correct the original picture (pull out the knife, untie the rope, surround the heat with ice, etc.) Use your imagination to "feel" instant improvement. You may be surprised to find how you can control pain in this way. (But remember that this should not be used as a substitute for appropriate medical attention.)

Recalling memories of particularly soothing scenes from your past is also quite useful. Involve as many of your senses as possible in visualizing your healing environment. Participate in the scene as completely as possible, by imagining the appropriate sights, sounds, smells, which feel most conducive to relaxation, peace, and contentment. Once you choose your health-affirming image for yourself, practice visualizing it as often as possible: in deep meditation, and many other times in your day, with the sense of patient expectation which, in religious terms, is known as faith.

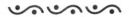

IX.

MEDITATION AND HEALTH

Although numerous methods may be employed... healing occurs primarily in consciousness.   —*Stephen Levine*

Due to some similarities and over-lapping uses, meditation and visualization have sometimes been taken as synonymous. Though they may seem like similar activites to the casual observer, they really constitute two different modes of consciousness. The distinction ought to be preserved so that beginners will be encouraged to investigate the value of working directly with consciousness in ways that only serious, traditional meditational practices can offer.

In visualization, mental events are actively generated for specific purposes, healing or otherwise. In meditation, attention is either fixed on one object, or mindfully attentive to the general contents of awareness, but no attempt is made to alter those contents. In fact, meditation has sometimes been described as "intentional purposelessness." The idea is to quiet the mind's incessant image/thought processing and perceive a clearer space behind it. This is a key difference between the two interior approaches. Visualization involves the directing of the symbolic, emotional, or conceptual powers of the mind, utilizing them creatively. Formal meditation is the stilling of mental processes—actually a different order of awareness. Visualization is something we *do.* Meditation is a way of being aware.

Both modes have demonstrated great potential in autonomous healing, and they are naturally compatible. The question of which method or combination is indicated for which diseases is an excellent one, worthy of future investigations. And it may be that, aside from the diagnostic variables, different types of people will have different aptitudes for each method. This helps make the case for the necessity of a teacher, but many self-starters can do well without one.

Meditation is: Turning inward. Quieting the mind. Opening perception. A way of centering and balance. Coming into the present. A source of inspiration and intuition. A tool for self-inquiry and discovery. Intrinsic freedom. Deepening and/or expanding awareness. It is *not* an escape from life's problems and the responsibility to act. It is not a religion.

The literature on healing abounds with references to the all-important "wholeness" experience, expressing it variously as homeostasis, unity, at-one-ment, integration, etc. In biology, no more direct analogy to this event exists than the effects of meditation on the human brain. It facilitates functional integration of the hemispheres, as evidenced in unusually synchronous brainwave activity ("hypersynchrony"), blood flow, and electrical potential distribution. Meditation allows for voluntary self-induction of the receptive alpha and theta brain wave states associated with heightened brain functioning.

Neurologically, meditation immediately and measureably alters brain chemistry and metabolism, increasing its oxygen supply by as much as 60% (even though overall consumption is reduced), releasing endorphins, and allowing a reconciliation between the cerebral cortex, which is the conscious, socialized part of the brain, and the diencephalon, the primitive, instinctual, subconscious part. Quite often these are at odds, due to the unnatural stress placed on the nervous system by our "civilized" way of living. When these parts of ourselves are brought into harmony through meditation, we are no longer fighting ourselves. We feel whole. In general, the practice dampens and even reverses the effects of negative stress, and rests all systems and organs in the body. Benefits of intermediate to long-term practice (several months to years) can be expected to include psychological as well as physical health improvements, including increased clarity of mind, receptivity, and learning capacities.

Meditation helps muscles, nerves, and the circulatory, digestive, hormonal and respiratory systems as well. It increases hemoglobin counts and reduces cholesterol in the blood. Since habits of breathing and posture play an important role in meditation, structural and organ re-alignment can also result, enhancing one's over-all appearance and well-being.

Because of his or her increased internal (proprioceptive) awareness, a meditator has a better chance of noticing unusual, pathological developments and correcting them earlier than a non-meditator. This is especially useful for onset prevention of migraine headaches, asthma attacks, and high blood pressure. The ability to meditatively psycho-locate specific organs within one's body is also valuable in cancer visualization therapy.

On the mental/emotional level, meditation is now acknowledged as a valid therapeutic modality for anxiety, depression, and other non-specific psychological syndromes, often as an adjunct therapy to biofeedback and counseling. Typical positive results include: alleviation of paranoia and aggression, greater sense of peace, more confidence and social ease, and more patience, optimism, and humor. The only contra-indications for meditation are schizophrenia, mental obsession, and other severe psychotic disorders.

Aside from the immediate curative and preventive benefits, the practice of meditation also facilitates high-level wellness and longevity. It can significantly enhance such higher faculties as memory, intuition and creativity. Other types of benefits attributed to meditation include greater self-esteem, more energy, better communication, and the feeling of joy that comes from achieving a higher level of awareness in one's life.

Spiritually, meditation is often reported as a catalyst for greater insight into one's purpose and role in life, a sense of unity and connectedness, and an understanding of the meaning of one's problems and pains. Often meditation becomes the doorway to a source of inner strength and guidance. It can be a significant help to people facing catastrophic illness and death.

APPROACHES TO MEDITATION

There is now an unprecedented amount of information available about the science of meditation. However, it should be obvious that infinitely more important than reading, discussing, and theorizing about meditation is the actual experience, the product of practice. Meditation is 99% commitment. My advice to any one seriously drawn to it is to set aside the time *every day* and simply begin sitting. If the dedication is there, the practice itself will lead towards growth. Meditation is not based on authority; it is a realization of one's own innate capacities.

As mentioned earlier, one of the most universally recommended practices for developing a meditative mind is "following the breath." Other objects of awareness used in various meditation systems include mandalas (concentric designs), flowers and candles (real and imagined), and the general contents of thought as it arises. In all these approches, the same single goal is the simple yet initially difficult achievement of complete and constant mindfulness.

The newcomer is confronted with a baffling array of styles of meditation to choose from, each with a different emphasis and perspective. There are focused meditations, with "objects," both external and internal, such as candle flame, or one's breath. There are visualizations, devotional practices, and color and healing meditations. There is also "empty," objectless meditation, which develops faculties of mindfulness, bare attention, and insight. And one can also meditate on subjects, usually metaphysical, such as levels of reality, or positive qualities of being. The list of traditional and innov-

innovative techniques is long, and it is up to the beginner to discern which he or she feels most affinity with through inner guidance, exposure to traditions, teachers, and books.

We can make a few general statements about how a beginner's path might unfold, by distilling out the most universal elements of meditation. Primary among these is the ingredient of body relaxation. In all the instructions that follow, it will be assumed that the reader has the ability to establish a working level of ease and physical comfort. Of course it will help to wear loose clothing, be relatively empty in the digestive tract, do a few basic stretches prior to the session, and sit in an upright, balanced posture.

After physical relaxation, most meditations involve some form of deliberate focusing. We could use the term "concentration" so long as it doesn't imply knitting one's brow and getting a headache. We are speaking of a very natural, uncomplicated act of pure attention. Call it "centering."

As mentioned, the most common focal point for developing the necessary meditative concentration is the breath. Another is the use of a "mantra," a repeated phrase (described further on). The idea is to sharpen and apply one's attention at will and to minimize the influence of distractions, including unrelated thoughts. With this ability to focus comes fresh kinds of awareness, and a certain degree of increased energy. It is primarily what is done with this energy that accounts for the diversity of meditative paths. For example, one can use it for healing, for religious devotion, for contemplating the wisdom of great teachers or books, for developing positive qualities, such as patience, generosity, and compassion. When concentration and energy are developed, there is no reason why one couldn't investigate all these approaches.

Ultimately, the specific meditative tools you will most rely upon will be determined by the type of person you are, and your particular needs. Give each one you try a good chance, then trust your intuition and follow your heart. And be open to change. (To avoid confusion and doubt, it is

important to discuss the dynamics of one's personal meditation practice only with qualified teachers or sincerely
interested spiritual friends. To talk of these matters casually
with those of limited commitment tends to devalue and
devitalize the experience.)

USEFUL ATTITUDES TO CULTIVATE:

*Cultivate moderation, equanimity, compassion, reverence, respect,
gratitude, simplicity, modesty, patience, and perseverance.*

A good teacher will caution you against going into
meditation for unusual experiences, or preconceived results.
Trying to "get" something, even health, is a dualistic mental
trap which perpetuates attachment and precludes satisfaction
and peace. Meditation is not petitionary prayer. Though the
"side effects" of meditation are often desirable and healthy,
freedom means having no expectations. Enlightenment is
natural mind. While meditating, we can simply notice all our
preconceptions, desires and attachments just as we would
any other capricious thoughts that might pop into the head.
Don't try to get any place where you're not. No demands, no
disappointments. Meditate mostly for the satisfaction of it,
and occasionally for no reason at all.

Meditation is deep but alert relaxation... seeing more
clearly... getting to know the inner Self... dropping your
usual concerns, or putting them in a more "cosmic"
perspective... getting "out of the body," or very into it!...
connecting, coming home... becoming pure energy, light...
being real.

MEDITATION AND THE INTELLECT

Meditation allows us to get beyond the limitations of our
rational, logical, deductive, and analytical faculties, making
room for spontaneous intuition and non-linear understanding
to come through. Yet ultimately, the brain-modes of intellect
and intuition are not mutually exclusive. Ideally, meditation
integrates all our faculties, and denies none. Avoid absolute
identification with any *one* mental capacity, and be free to

choose any as appropriate to the moment. There's no reason why meditation shouldn't satisfy one's quest for knowledge as well as one's search for peace. Just remember that there's a difference between *seeing* and *being.* Ultimately the intellect cannot grasp non-duality, wherein one is no longer meditating *on* something, but rather there is just consciousness itself, unattached and unencumbered.

AFTER-EFFECTS

The after-effects of meditation vary from person to person and from session to session. One person might leave a sitting with an over-abundance of energy, while another might be so calmed down as to not wish to move at all. You may find, after meditating for some time, that you require less sleep. The practice has also been known to affect people's dream life in various ways.

Meditation can also tend to reinforce or magnify any of our usual propensities and habits, particularly at the early stages. Thus, for example, if you are a very sensuous person, you may feel more hungry or lustful after meditating. Intellectual types might want to read or write more. Altruistic people will feel even more generous. In general, it's most useful to do something creative with the energy generated in meditation, rather than leave it unexpressed, bottled up, so to speak.

BEGIN. Regularity of practice is most important, especially at the beginning. Start with a short session every morning (sunrise is ideal*). It should soon become a pleasant enough experience that duration and frequency grow naturally, but excuses for procrastination are bound to test your motivation. You may have to exert more self-control and discipline to deepen the practice. Later, your meditation may become a kind of positive addiction, which you will definitely miss when you skip a session or two.

---

* An additional evening session is most beneficial. You will discover a different quality of meditative experience at different times of day.

An occasional formal extended retreat can create an excellent foundation for a new practice, or re-establish an old one. In any case, try to sit daily, no matter how briefly. In this way, a strong, deep and reliable meditative practice is made from hundreds of modest affirmations of intent. Meditation is a commitment to the best in you.

The most important first step is setting aside the time in your daily routine. As soon as you can, simply sit down in a quiet place and "go within." Take a few moments to find your center of gravity. Relax, and get still. Soon the process will begin to feed and heal you.

RITUAL

Ritual can be an intelligent and inspiring use of familiarity for self-inducing the Relaxation Response, higher states of mind, and healing. Any activity associated with these positive states, repeated regularly, can become a useful ritual. Examples include lighting candles and incense, chanting, and symbolic movement. Other options for ritual include: consecrations, offerings, invocations, affirmations, and vows.

Rituals should not be done automatically, for their own sake. That's like going to a restaurant and eating the menu. If a ritual is not executed consciously, and fails to create the awareness it was originally associated with, then it has outlived its usefulness. Design your own meditation/healing ritual and invest it with meaning, so that whenever you return to it, it will be a potent reminder of your higher purposes.

For purification, symbolic and actual cleansing rituals are an important part of spiritual and healing meditation. Each time, before starting, purify yourself (in body, speech and thought) and your place of meditation. Repetition of this detail will reveal its significance and power.

HELPFUL HINTS

Some hints are: a quiet setting, soft lighting, comfortable clothing, empty stomach, upright and balanced posture, relaxed muscles, regularity and ritual. Also, perseverance with humor. Have no expectations and take your time.

RELAXATION. Deliberately and systematically let go of the tension in each part of the body, from the top down, particularly on successive exhalations. Use positive auto-suggestive thoughts (such as "I am whole," "Peace is Here," etc.), or images of peaceful surroundings.

Sometimes just being still will constitute the first difficulty in meditation. When the urge to move arises, breathe out tension. A funny paradox is that once you get to a certain depth of body awareness, you may also feel "out of the body," and stillness becomes natural, while movement seems like effort.

LETTING GO. Aside from muscle tension you can voluntarily let go of mental anxiety, fear, anger, guilt and unworthiness, desires, preconceptions, poor self-image, and negative personality traits. Even thoughts can be dropped, resulting in a pleasant experience of spaciousness and freedom from agitation. Allow yourself the feelings suggested by these words: *Open. Trust. Accept. Float. Surrender. Detach. Flow. Release. Give. Evaporate.* Do yourself a favor and read this paragraph again.

CENTERING. To minimize distractions and a scattered feeling, choose a focal point within your body/mind, such as the breath, heartbeat or one of the *chakras* (inner energy centers) such as the forehead center. Dwell on it with passive alertness. Use images of balance and depth. Create a *mandalla* (concentric design) in your mind. Be at the center.

MANTRAS

Mantras are special phrases or seed syllables which are repeated audibly or sub-vocally for concentration and empowerment. Traditional mantras are taken as sacred and used for inspiration (as with names or qualities of God), and for self-healing (e.g., autogenic phrases). Often the mantra is "invested" by a teacher, in an initiation ceremony, but this is not necessarily the only way to "receive" one. You can simply choose a mantra, or you can keep your inner ear open and wait for the universe to suggest one. Or invent your own. Here are some possibilities. Say each a few times in rhythm with your breathing, and see how they feel:

● English: *Toward the One. Be here now. Love is All. Know Me, God. I Am Light. This Too Shall Pass. Attention, witness, absorb, flow. All is well, all is one. Lord Jesus Christ have mercy on me. Let the light shine within and without. Be still and know I am. Peace above, peace below, peace all around, peace within. The power of God is within me, the love of God is all around.*
● Sanskrit: *Om* (Universal sound). *Ram* (Creator). *Shi-Vah* (Transformer). *AhNam* (The Nameless). *Kali* (Divine Mother). *Shanti* (Peace).
● Others: *Om Mani Padme Hum* (Tibetan, Jewel in the Lotus). *Om Ah Hum* (Tibetan, The power of all). *La ilaha illa llah* (Muslim, There is no God but God). *Alleluia* (Christian).

A particularly Buddhist approach uses no specific object of meditation at all. Instead, one simply notices with "bare attention" (Pali: *Satipathana:* "choiceless awareness") whatever sensation or mental event presents itself at any moment, with the intention of perceiving just what is actually present, clearly, and then letting it go. In this way, the reactivity, prejudice, and attachment of one's own mind become included as objects of meditative, dispassionate scrutiny. The keys to this method are keen alertness coupled with constantly renewed non-attachment, non-judgement, and non-reaction. Cultivate the mind of "active passivity."

ATTENTION & CONCENTRATION. An untrained mind is like a child at a carnival; it will stray and linger with whatever happens to grab its attention. Daydreaming is *not* meditation, no matter how correct one's posture may be. For this reason perserverance is required in continuously returning the mind to a center of clarity. This should be done repeatedly, with patience, gently and firmly, as a loving mother would train a child to stay out of traffic. It is neither necessary nor helpful to make a forceful confrontation with the wandering mind, as this tends to reinforce its resistance. Simply notice old habits, give them space, like clouds in the sky, and then carefully turn the attention to the desired focus. As in all worthwhile human endeavors, repeated practice will bring results.

ABOUT DROWSINESS. Quite often, and more so at the beginning of one's training in meditation, the necessary alertness will seem elusive. At such times it is quite easy to feel convinced that you are simply "too tired to meditate," but in most instances this will actually be false fatigue, a kind of psychological laziness, or resistance to change. In actuality, meditation is often more restful than a good "catnap." As an experiment, try not giving in to the first few impulses to quit. You may be pleasantly surprised to discover that a little discipline engenders a great deal of energy. Simply take a few deep breaths and renew your meditation with an attitude of sure determination. This will have the double benefit of deepening your practice and developing the power of good commitment.

CHANGES. Some people might avoid meditation for fear of becoming changed in some way, or losing control of their lives, perhaps because they have seen radical changes in people that joined various exotic religious groups. Private, non-institutionalized meditation requires no surrender to any authority or belief system outside one's self. It's more like looking in a mirror. Only those who have been hiding from themselves will be surprised, but they needn't be upset. Meditation allows us to flow through our necessary growth more gracefully, with greater understanding and less anxiety. Through it we become more authentic and cling less to a superficial self-image. All life involves change, but meditative changes usually seem more natural and timely.

X.

ANNE, A PERSONAL ACCOUNT

He who has a why to live, can bear most any how. —*Nietzsche*

I first met Anne at a cancer support group for which I was conducting a guided relaxation session at the request of the group's doctor. The most noticeable thing about her was her extreme difficulty in breathing, for she suffered from severe asthma. It took me a few moments to see past her obvious discomfort, but it soon became evident that Anne's spirit was very much intact. She emanated kindness and sincerity.

Anne called me for holistic health counseling, and yoga stretching and breathing instructions. When we met, she had just been through three of the most stressful life-changes on the Holmes and Rahe scale*: a divorce, a career change, and a home relocation. She was also struggling with a number of serious illnesses, including breast cancer, asthma, and emphysema. She had a long history of surgery including the removal of her tonsils, appendix, and ovaries.

At 52, Anne might have had sufficient reasons to despair about life, but she was far from defeated. One of the traits that

---

* Holmes, T.H. & R.H. Rahe. 1967. "Social Readjustment Rating Scale," *Journal of Psychosomatic Research.* November, pages 213-218.

people cannot help but notice in Anne is her spontaneous and prolific sense of humor.* I felt I could help her help herself.

Anne's initial consultation and questionnaires revealed that she could use assistance in areas of self-confidence, expressing feelings, personal goal setting, stress reduction, and diet.

Eventually the modalities we worked with included nutrition, biofeedback, meditation, guided imagery, and yoga. I recorded a relaxation tape for Anne, and she is presently enrolled in her third 8-week yoga course. Her efforts are inspiring and her progress continues to be very encouraging. She still periodically experiences acute respiratory distress, but says that the yoga deep breathing exercises help. Her cancer is in complete remission.

Anne is one of those whom Bernie Siegel calls the exceptional cancer patient. She fought back. Over the last year and a half I've had the privilege of watching her go through a rebirth and transformation. Her excitement about discovering new ways of seeing the world is wonderful to behold. Her enthusiasm is contagious. Sometimes it seems as if she's getting younger. Even if she had not succeeded in curing her cancer, she triumphed in terms of personal happiness and the quality of her life. Anne has found peace. Within that peace her commitment to living is total.

INTERVIEW WITH A SURVIVOR

The following is an interview I had with Anne in her home, discussing her experiences and insights as a veteran cancer patient.

---

* It is to Doctor Reid's credit that he has introduced so much laughter into the lives of his cancer group members. Humor is not only spiritually uplifting, but neuro-chemically healthy and stress-reducing too.[1]

Anne, what was the doctor's recommendation when they first discovered the cancer, chemotherapy?

Yes, the recommendation for follow-up treatment, in essence said that I had no more than a 15% chance.

Of living?

Yes, well, of having the chemotherapy cure me. So my daughter and I decided, why go through all that pain. That's not much of a bargain. We decided against it, prior to knowing of "self-healing," and (Dr. Reid)[2] and the Simontons and all of that . . .

You just decided to relax.

Well, not only that; I was right in the midst of the most trying part of the divorce. I was without a home, essentially, and one of my sons had just gotten married, which was a happy thing, but they do list that in the list of "life-traumas" that you go through.

So you think the divorce and life stresses were related to your illness?

Oh, absolutely no question in my mind! Definitely. I had had some lumps in both of my breasts, but I had monitored them with a doctor every six months, and at the very toughest time of the divorce it was time for another check-up. And I said I couldn't face it. Isn't it silly, that was the wrong one to let go by. And then I noticed that I had lymph node swelling.

So there was major crisis in every aspect of your life.

Yeah.

And the doctor said, basically, you had 15% chance of surviving.

Well that was the fellow who wanted to do the chemotherapy. He was very aggressive. Really a tough, tough man . . . I mean he was willing to sit there with me and explain everything until I ran out of questions, but he was not happy when I said I either wanted to think it over more, or talk it over, or I didn't want it. He didn't want to hear those things.

How does that make you feel?

Well, . . . angry. Because I don't know why he would want to put anyone through the obvious pain or discomfort, or whatever, of chemotherapy, for such a little bit of hope.

Well, of course his training is: If there's any chance of cure, you go for it, like you said, aggressively. To him, the more aggressive the better. That's his way of increasing the chances.

I felt very small, and very much as though what I felt made little or no difference. Have you ever been pulled over by a state trooper? Maybe they don't do that to men, but that just happened to me. It was because I didn't have my diesel sticker. So I said well, maybe it's on the front of the car, and the back one's come off or something. So he walked around and came back and he says, "No, there's just your handicap sticker, lady." Then I wanted to hit him.

But you didn't say anything.

No. I said, "Well, I guess I just have to pay the fine, how much will it be?" And he said, "Oh, around a hundred twenty-five dollars." And then I cried. And that shifted the weight a lot.

It's interesting that you compare your surgeon to a state trooper. Did you cry with the doctor?

Oh, yes. He said, "Why are you crying??!" Like that.

Real accusatory...?

Yeah.

Did your doctor give you an estimate of how long you had to live?

No, I didn't even read that paper till I got home. Oh, and if you really want to (share my anger) with me ... he and this whole troop marched into my room in the hospital and said, "I've discussed your case with so and so" (there were three of them there at the end of my bed), "and this is what we've determined." I said, well I'll have to think about that because I was right in the middle of a divorce, I was going to start to build a house, I didn't have a home, etc. You know what he said? "Well we can't concern ourselves with those things." And I think he really did me a favor when he said that.

Why?

Well, because if he wasn't concerned with that, *I'd* better darn well be! And in fact, I don't think I consciously understood this but, what you have to do is gather all the facts and then you are responsible for your own health. Even before any of this happened, I always believed that.

It's incredible the way they try to deny that: "Here's what we've decided." When he said "we can't concern ourselves with that"... that's the opposite of holistic.

That's like saying, "Lady, you're responsible for everything but your chemotherapy, and that's what we're gonna do for you." Maybe someday I'll make an appointment and just go chat with him.

Write him a letter.

I might do that. I was going to wait 'till I had gotten past the point of having to hit him, and then maybe I could *enlighten* him!

You could enlighten a lot of people.

Well, I've got to get my act together first. Get a little stronger.

You're getting there.

Oh, yeah, well, I'm going in the right direction, but as a basically impatient person, I am learning to move a lot slower and still be encouraged by it. 'Cause everything in my life always had to be yesterday, you know? That was the way I walked. Everything. Darted everywhere. Or else just collapsed. Not much in between.

So, there you were, pretty devastated...

Yeah, and then the asthma hit. That was the end of July.

Was that new?

Brand new. I had respiratory emphysema. But the inflammation of the upper respiratory tract was brand new. So maybe I didn't get the message with the cancer, huh?

Well, there's several messages. I really think asthma has a lot to do with unexpressed feelings. Rage... grief.

Yes.

And the cancer, it happened just when you were going from wife and mother and successful business-person to divorcee and retired and alone.

How depressing!

Well it's interesting that you use that word, because mental/emotional depression also depresses your immune system, and that's when cancer cells can multiply.

That's good, I never thought of that.

The Simontons point that out. Chemically, clinically, this is verifiable with blood counts. People who are grieving or despairing, who have gone through major loss, are at greater risk for immune system diseases. Including cancer.

Well, maybe I've licked it.

Well, you've gone from giving up on your life to a great sense of enthusiasm.

True.

You know, cancer can function as a socially acceptable form of suicide.

And it's the most dramatic of all diseases; it's sort of the one thing that's an instant message to the rest of the world.

In your case, what was that message?

... Love me. *(Here, Anne cries.)*

It's a cry for help.

And I've received a lot of help. My heart's very full... We must all love each other.

I know. It's good for our health!

Well, it's just another dimension. Because life could really be kind of a drag. I mean I don't get off on scrubbing floors or washing windows... and I really hate to vacuum! But love makes it worthwhile. Forgive me, I'm still somewhat apologetic about crying, because it was certainly nothing that was ever acceptable in my youth... (pause)

... What happened after your diagnosis? You declined treatment.

Really with the help of my daughter. She said, "Don't put yourself through that." Driving to Boston and all that. At this point I had the asthma. It just wasn't worth the odds. She helped me make the wisest choice.

It probably saved your life, even though at the time you thought you were turning down the only possible treatment.

You know, I've got good kids. When I was dying, it was my

thoughts of them that made the difference. I thought, if my ex-husband really is as bad as I think he is, it's really not nice of me to die and leave him these children that are in this great turmoil going round and round, with no apparent thing to grab onto. So in essence that's the only thing that motivated me.

You found a reason to live!

Yeah. That's when I quit smoking, because I knew I had respiratory problems, and I thought, well it's worth a try. And I want to just see if I can get them a little more organized and together.

That was a really conscious decision!

Oh, definitely.

Were you just sort of lying in bed one night and you thought it all out, and that's what you realized!

I think it was from a real sense of responsibility. I've always had a very strong sense of responsibility.

So to die would have been irresponsible to your children!

Yeah, will it would be a real dirty trick. I mean if in fact I really believed this about my husband. I understand him a whole lot better now, and I'm a lot less "black and white" about him, but in fact he is not necessarily a "natural parent."

That's a diplomatic way of saying it.

Whatever his whole . . . you know, condition was, he took it out on the children. I guess all this led to the feeling that if I really feel this way about him, then step two is: You don't just die, or you don't just quit. It was conscious. 'Cause they had two parents, and I was the other one.* This was at the end of the marriage. When I knew there was no way to save it. No way to put it back together. I think that's where things started to change. Can you have a nervous breakdown without being diagnosed?

Oh, sure. Clearly you got psychologically exhausted.

---

* Anne has referred several times to this important realization in reference to her recovery: that she could fulfill her role as an equal parent (instead of subordinate to the father), gave her a renewed will to live.

That's it. No place left to turn.

So you almost turned off, is what you're saying.

Uh huh.

But it was the thought of your kids having to be under your husband's control, without you there, that made you want to rescue them, in a way.

Yes, stay afloat a little longer.

And that was a decisive realization, or moment, and things kind of changed from there?

Yes. Maybe I didn't do it soon enough, but still in all, I know it's sort of trite and today everyone's talking about it, but I really feel cancer was sort of a gift, or a message. Maybe that's not unique with me but I think it's fact. I agree with it.

The fact that you can say that is very significant.

I had a woman friend who used to work with me, who's been a problem to me off and on, and has re-entered my life when she heard about the cancer, and did it in a very aggressive way. Anyway she called me last night because I wrote her, and I said that I really was a happy person, and she kept challenging me: "How can you be?" And I said, "If cancer did that for me, then I am grateful." Cancer. People have difficultly with it. I don't mean having cancer, but having a friend who has it.

You become a symbol of their fears.

And you're somewhat of a threat because, if they're too nice to you, you might become their responsiblity, you know. Watson says cancer turns up your burners. So I am in fact more sensitive, but in a way I'm much less sensitive than I used to be. Anyway, my friend said that the letter I sent her was so beautiful she took it and read it to her friends. I thought, oh my God, I ripped that off in about five minutes. So maybe I am here to give messages. Cancer made me put my brakes on. It made me stop and think about things, which I don't think the divorce would have done. The divorce was just another rejection, or failure.

I bet you don't feel like a failure now.

No, I guess I haven't thought about it that much, but I

don't feel success or failure.

You're no longer measuring it.

Yeah. One of the neat things yoga did for me was: There's no success or failure in yoga because you just do what you're able to, and then a little more. And another thing I've learned: Somehow I grew up with the idea that if you wanted to do something you tried it, and if it didn't work, then obviously it wasn't for you. And that is so unfortunately simplistic. Somehow I have given you credit for teaching me: If it doesn't work the first time then you try it more than once! *(Laughs.)* So I'm back for more, because I really do want to succeed.

In yoga as in life!

I don't know whether you mean to give off these messages, but I'm sure I'm not the only one receiving them.

Well, it's like you didn't mean to cry in front of the State Trooper. It just happens.

There's a lot of electricity in that yoga room. I mean good stuff! I get it all the way over here, just getting into the car!

Great! Pretty soon you won't even have to get into the car: just tune in psychically, and save gas!

Oh, and there are times when I've ended in tears after your meditation. I take my glasses off so I go out of focus, just so everything is softer, and then I put my glasses on, and mine aren't the only wet eyes. I think there are a lot of people out there who need that. I think we're just coming to that. I feel, aren't I lucky to be alive now. I don't mean that "cancer-wise," I mean in this time, this generation... *(pause)*

... So let's continue... You got the diagnosis, and you decided not to go for chemotherapy, and you didn't get radiation, and you were pretty much in "the dark night of your soul" there.

Yes.

What happened?

I read a little article, a little square this big, in the *Milford Cabinet*, about Dr. Watson Reid, speaking at the "Y" in Nashua.

One of those cosmic coincidences.

Oh, I can really "get off" on that one. I said to Keith, my son, would you go with me? and he said sure. We got there late and there were only two seats left, right in the front row, under Watson's nose! And somebody there brought up Bernie Siegel...

What was the topic of the talk, Cancer and Psychotherapy?

Yes, it was the Simonton approach to cancer. And then it had a flyer about his (cancer patients support) group.

And you went.

Oh, definitely. I'll tell you, I just remembered something that isn't as prominent in my mind as it was then, but for some reason I wanted—I was *driven*, would be a fair word—to be with other cancer people. And I never figured that out. I really stopped trying to, I guess.

It's the power of support.

Maybe I expected instant understanding or something.

Well you wouldn't be a pariah, an outcast.

Yes, or, "What the hell did you do that for, dummy?"

Blame.

Yeah. I guess I wanted more information. I love information. So then Keith and I went on to Bernie Siegel's lecture. At the end, Keith said to me, "Oh, yeah, that's how I got rid of my warts!" And I said, *"What?"* This kid really hates any pain of any sort, and he did this at college, when it was time to come home at Christmas and get more needles. It isn't that I didn't believe him, I just found it very weird. At the end, when the meditation came, Keith said, "If I fall asleep, just punch me, 'cause I usually do." So I guessed he'd been doing this somewhere before.

So the whole approach was essentially about the power of the mind?

Yes. Oh, and this whole experience with imagery, and the children's drawings, and the whole message. So I'm certain that just Keith's being so natural about the whole thing was a big help to me, just like my daughter saying "Don't even think about chemotherapy!"

Boy, she may have saved your life.

Oh, I know she did. Oh definitely.

... by telling you to believe in something bigger than the medical establishment.

She didn't even believe in mastectomies. We used to call them "Mistakes to me!" I wrote that to my surgeon, on our first anniversary (of surgery). By the time I got back to him, I don't know whether he chose to ignore it, or whether I was just #302 or something like that, but he never mentioned it. However I'm certain mine was at a point that...

You needed it...

Well, I guess I can't say that, but I hadn't even heard of any "mind-over-matter" kind of alternatives at that point.

What was the first meeting at Watson's support group like? Or the first time you really felt like you were on to something?

Oh, well I had read the (Simonton's) book. And thought, wait a minute, here are more of these...woo...

Cosmic connections...?

Yeah, right! Oh I loved it! Well you know for the little merchant who sells broken furniture, this was a whole new experience to me! I mean, "wait a minute, here... OK, I'll try to remain open, but if somebody didn't plan this..."uh, you know.

That's exciting.

Yes it was. So the first meeting was a mind blower. I had never been in a family or group experience where people would just stand up and say, "I've had half of my brain removed, and I can't see the roads, and they won't let me drive anymore." You know, I mean I couldn't even say where my cancer *was.* I just said I'm Anne from Amherst, and I'm a cancer person.

So you got the company of other cancer patients, which you wanted. It's been important to you, I take it. You're still going?

Oh yeah. This is after a year and half.

You must have lost a few members in that time?

Yes...I'm very interested in death.

So am I.

I mean if we can talk about sex and all those other good things...

Death is the last taboo.

Maybe we all just move out to the next ring around us.

Everything in its time, huh? I read once, "Until you face death you can't face life." Or do I have that backwards?

Well, it makes sense both ways!

Oh good! That's even more important now. I like that. You know we can't even get (the topic of death) cranked up in the cancer support group. Maybe that's what I'm there for.

What do you do there, visualizations, relaxation techniques?

Yes. And I'm a very visual person, and I think that must help. Things make pictures for me.

Did you immediately believe in the methods used in this kind of therapy?

Yes. I didn't know whether *step one* would make *step two* a certainty, but I was more than willing to do *step one.* Whether it would get rid of, or ward off, cancer, I didn't *not* believe, but I guess I didn't just buy the whole package right off. But I certainly thought that whole Simonton approach had great merit.

Did you deal with goal setting?

Yes. Goals I found difficult. Because I guess I had been sort of—or thought of myself as—a "non-person" person. One time I remember saying that I could walk past a mirror without creating an image.

Like feeling empty of identity?

Yeah, just sort of wafting around, without... a sense of myself.

Was building your house part of your "goal setting," or was it just something that you had to do out of necessity?

Well, I don't know. I received a settlement and had to have a place to live, but what I've always loved was land. Helen (Anne's astrologer friend) tells me I'm a very "earth" person. Plus I think it meant to me a continuation of "home" as far as children were concerned. I designed it, and the kids all contributed their thoughts. I said "OK, you guys all tell me what color you want your room." The painter said, "I gotta meet this family!"... You know cancer does shorten your "distant view" of life. Which is good.

You stopped postponing becoming who you really are.

Maybe it's when you realize that something is going to be taken away, or *could* be. You really look at it. And appreciation can come from that.

And you cried a lot?

Yes, that was good. And anger, I knew I had to work that out with (her ex-husband). I'm not really angry at him any more. However, there are times I'd like to let the air out of his tires ! I don't want to kill him now, but I like to give him a little bit of a problem ! *(we laugh)*

It seems like a balance between being honest about your anger and forgiving.

Well one would have to precede the other.

The Simontons point out that the more honest you are about your anger, the less chance there is for storing resentment. I guess the trick is to allow yourself to feel anger without trying to hurt anybody with it.

Well, I always hated my temper, because I hated my father's temper. But now I realize that temper and anger are not necessarily together. You can be angry with *conditions,* but you don't have to strike out at another human being.

(We then talked of how Anne was progressively introduced to some of the concepts and practices of self-healing, including yoga, natural diet & supplements.)

What did you change in your diet?

Well a year ago I started giving up meat and animal fats. I was a big cheese eater. I don't know whether it's just that, or that and yoga together, but I lost around 10 pounds. But now I hear more and more about diet and cancer. I think somebody needs to blow the whistle.

When did you realize you were completely free of cancer? When did you see the doctor?

Well, I go every three months. It takes him about 90 seconds to check me out. This is the surgeon, so what can he tell me, unless he sees a lump or something? He just looks at his handiwork and that's it. One time I pasted a heart there, you know the ones the kids stick on the back of their envelopes ! *(much laughter)*

So, did the doctor concur that you had improved?

Well you know I recently had to have intestinal surgery for a blockage, and I said, OK, well while you're in there, if you're anywhere near the liver, would you take a look, because there was still a "shadow" that came up on the CAT scan. And so the guy did, and he said, there's absolutely nothing wrong. He said there's a little surface irregularity but nothing like what we thought. The other "shadow" was here, under my sternum, and those are both gone.

Anne, what did your whole experience with cancer mean to you, or do for you?

Cancer really helped give me a control of my life that I don't think I've had. I don't mean initially, because at the time it happened to me I was totally out of control of my life. But I think that dealing with it made me gain more control. I think it gave me permission, like sort of a blank ticket, to perhaps do all the things you've always wanted to do, and you didn't have enough self-confidence or togetherness or whatever to do them for yourself; or to allow yourself to do them.

So now you had the greatest excuse in the world: You were dying.

Yes, that's it. I mean it is a universal buzz word that everybody understands. I think there are people with diseases that I probably have never heard of and couldn't pronounce, that are perhaps suffering far more, but cancer, everybody knows what that is ... whether what we all feel about cancer is right or wrong. I mean there are more deaths from heart disease, but cancer is much more of a bugaboo word. A bogey man kind of thing.

It's true, it's got a stigma to it, but at the same time you could use that as a ticket to freedom. In other words, people couldn't blame you now for doing anything, because you had cancer.

You know they say in "self-healing," pick something you've always wanted to do, and for God's sakes go about doing it. And I thought and thought, and said I don't think I really have a goal. But I decided I've always wanted to go to Europe by boat. So I started to get that all together, and it just didn't have any meaning for me. It just sort of dissolved. But after I'd been in therapy with Dr. Reid for a while, I realized, "This is what I've always wanted to do!"

Therapy?

Well, that's sort of a cocktail word, but you know I just wanted a lot of answers. Always wanted a lot of answers, and I didn't know whether going back to school would have done it or what, but it turned out that through things that people suggested I read, one door led to another door and another.

Learning. Self-discovery, which you probably wouldn't have given yourself permission to do before you got sick.

No. Several times I've tried to go back to school, and I got the brochure from the State University, and it said "Psychology I & II," and I said, oh I can't take that. I didn't think I was qualified. Not some little housewife going back to school, you know? Take a course in "American Literature," 'cause that's what your son studied, and then you can talk better with him; you know that kind of thing. And so that's all I signed up for. *Now,* looking back on that, I think how far I've grown past that point.

That was before your diagnosis?

Yeah. I was kind of intimidated by the world.

And now you've outgrown that? If you wanted to take a psychology course, you would.

Oh definitely.

In fact, you're probably very qualified!

I'd take a "Pre-Med" course now if I wanted to, because I know I'm not hurting anyone and that I have that right as much as the next person. *That* I think is something non-obvious that cancer did for me. And we talked about receiving love and care and I'm certain that *that* all played a part in the benefits of cancer. It's kind of a self-respect I think you learn. Just basic. Just because you are a human being. Not because you're a special human being, but just for the fact that you were created and born and you exist.

Well that didn't always sound so obvious before. You were born and existed and deserved love, but you didn't always let yourself feel it.

Oh, no. And that's very exciting to me.

Did you feel more love because people knew you had cancer, or did you feel more love because you finally let yourself let it in?

I've thought about that a lot, and I don't know whether you can really separate them. Because probably it was already always there, don't you suppose? I do. I think it was probably always there, I mean all the same people that now I feel love me were always part of my life. I think cancer, or I suppose any trauma, opens you to a deeper level of sensitivity to what's going on around you. You know Al, in our group, always says he smells more flowers and sees more sunsets. Cancer just sort of steps the pace back a little. Slows you down. So much doesn't just rush past you.

Sounds great! It should happen to everybody!

It certainly helped me get a sense of self-worth. That's something I guess I've never had. The other thing is that it gave me a sense of, "If you're going to get it together, you'd better get at it!" A little time compression.

You stopped procrastinating.

Yeah, or saying, well someday I'd like to learn about this or that or have a better relationship with my older son, or whatever. It gives you a sense of today-ness. Immediacy. Cancer was like a dart on the board. Like a bolt. You know with this respiratory thing I've had three operations in the last year, and I'm a very high risk for dying under anesthesia. So you're glad to wake up. You feel you've been given another shot at it. Three times! I think you say to yourself, well hell, you'd better make use of it. Plus an awareness of death. You sort of want to neaten up your life. Helen said, "Whatever light is around you at the time, you take with you and is yours." There's that: looking a little bit beyond just today, too.

Do you have any major goals now?

Yes, I would like to return something to the world. And I'm not sure what that is, but it's like when I realized how just a phone call from a friend had really helped me out, I thought, there must be somebody else out there.

Pass it on.

Yeah, I did. It was wonderful. It was so much fun! I thought, well now, if I called two people, and they were affected in a similar manner, they might each call two people, and—you know I have this wonderful imagination—in two weeks everybody could be happy! Anyway, I thought, if you don't know what to do, but if you give to others what you enjoy receiving, then at least you can do that much. Do you know how many people are really grateful to receive a card in the mail? And not necessarily sick people.

Do you have any advice for others going through the same thing? What would you tell a friend who just received a diagnosis of cancer?

I would offer help . . . Gee I never thought about that. It's not easy. Because "self-healing" or whatever name you want to put on it, I think, involves a hard look at yourself. (Anne is crying at this point.)

It's OK.

And you may need help doing that. I know *I* did. Because you can't always see as clearly as someone else can, especially a trained someone else. Then, I think the hard look comes first, and probably the second thing that has to happen is change. And I think a hell of a lot of people, and I'm one of them, find change very difficult.

Making changes?

Oh, yeah, you fight it terribly.

Changing your habits? character?

Your lifestyle, whatever.

It's hard work.

Well you remember what happened when Bernie Siegel mailed out several hundred invitations to cancer patients.

Yeah, he got twelve responses.

I think that's very significant.

Human nature resists change.

Yes. You know how when an aerialist has to let go of one swing before they grab the other . . . and there's that moment when you're hanging out there all alone. Where you simply can't have any guarantees.

It's a leap of faith.

Well, I think if those two things are involved: the real deep look inside, and then . . . maybe from that not everyone makes the next step, or changes, but certainly that's what I gathered from it.

I think the ability and the desire to make the change increases your chances of recovery.

Yes. I'm not really thinking so much of recovery. Just today. Quality of life.

But I think you're right, that a certain percentage, maybe even a majority of people who are that sick give up, at that point, when they can't face making those changes. In a way, it's easier to be lazy.

Yeah, and I'm going to have to do it again. Well, if cancer returns . . . All of this wonderful stuff I've been saying, I'm going to have to practice.

But don't you do that every day?

Well, yeah, I do, I guess. But anyway, just because I think I've sort of worked it out for myself, I'm not certain it's what I could guarantee anyone else. It seems to me you give somebody tools with which to work. I mean you can't leave them with much else. *(Anne is crying.)*

This is all still hard for you, I know. Why does it make you cry, do you know?

No. And I've given up worrying about it, 'cause I cry so much! I used to worry, but now I just let it pour out. Maybe I'll dehydrate to death *(laughs).*

It's cleansing.

I'm just catching up. I was never allowed to cry. It was, "you're a sissy, a baby, " you know, all that crap.

Someone once said "Never miss an opportunity to cry."

That's nice. And then if you don't fight it, then it only happens when it has to, as opposed to . . . all other times.

Anne, are you still taking Prednisone?

Yes, as an anti-inflammatory for the bronchial tract. But I've been thinking about that, and I haven't been as diligent about imagery in that area as I was imaging the cancer, and I don't think I'm using all of my potential in that regard.

You mean you have a feeling you could taper off the Prednisone?

Oh, there's no question. I've already done that. I'm way down to 2½ milligrams a day, from 40 or 60 in the hospital, a year ago. And I had flu in April, and I had to go up again. You can jump up in dosage, but not down. You have to wean yourself.

You have withdrawal symptoms if you don't?

That's what they say. I've never tried it, but they all warn you not to.

But in the long term you're anticipating tapering off?

That's my goal, yes. You see Prednisone makes you cookoo. It makes you hyper, jittery. But this is where the yoga comes in. It's in direct relation to the amount of yoga I'm doing. The next step is 2½ milligrams every *other* day. And the doctor said, "Don't ever try to take none." Well that's all he had to tell me, 'cause that's my goal, of course! Anyway I think yoga is toning up my body. And it's making better use of what I got. Whether yoga is going to cure my ills or not is really unimportant; it's going to give me the greatest potential for doing that. You see, as soon as the body just sags, then all the strain goes into the respiratory system.

You've felt that?

Oh, no question.

So you really directly link your condition with your yoga practice?

Oh, definitely. There's no question. The time I felt the very best was when you taught 16 weeks in a row. At the end of that was when I got down to taking Prednisone every other day.

How are you doing with alcohol?

Good. I have a little wine in the evening. Sometimes not. You know I used to drink a fair amount of scotch. My life used to be pretty "cocktailly."

Was it hard to change that?

No. It just didn't taste good after a while. And of course alcohol is a depressant not only emotionally, but it depresses the whole respiratory system. So it just makes the breathing harder.

So you don't want it?

Right.

Well I don't have any more questions. Do you have anything else to say?

Just that I love you!

I love you too, Anne.

CHART CAPTIONS

I. TWO HEALTH PARADIGMS
Compares health care premises and approaches of conventional (allopathic) and alternative (holistic) medical philosophies.

2. THE ILLNESS/WELLNESS CONTINUUM
Depicts the range of states of health encompassed by holism.

3. THE HOLISTIC SPECTRUM OF INTERVENTION
This chart shows the variety of interventions classified by types and ordered by degrees of severity: Toward the left of the spectrum are those healing modalities that are most self-sufficient, preventive, low-tech, low-risk, inexpensive, and natural.

4. THE CIRCLE OF HEALTH FACTORS
Shows the influences on human health, as slices in a pie.

5. OPTIMUM HEALTH FACTORS
This is an overview of positive health influences in a person's life, and related obstacles.

6. HIGH-LEVEL WELLNESS
Some attributes of optimum health from the holistic perspective.

Two Health Paradigms

ALLOPATHIC	HOLISTIC
Focuses on: Symptoms Measurements	Focuses on: Causes & Patterns Feelings
Disease as Entity — Pain-avoiding General Classified Diagnosis	Pain-Reading — Disease as Process Specific Atypical Needs
Technical Tools	*Integrated Therapies*
Remedial Combative Reactive	Preventive Corrective Pro—active
Crisis Oriented Occasional Intervention Radical. Defensive.	Lifestyle Oriented Sustained Maintenance Natural. Ecological.
Side-Effects — MEDICINE As Counter-Agent Iatrogenesis Chemicals—Surgery—Radiation	MEDICINE As Co-Agent — Low—Risk Conservative Organic Purification—Manipulation—Release
Emphasis: "CURE" Speed. Comfort. Convenience.	Emphasis: "HEALING" Homeostasis. Restoration Regeneration. Transformation
Practitioner as Authority *Pacifying* Patient as Passive Recipient	Practitioner as Educator *Activating* Patient as Source of Healing
Mechanical/Analytical *Bio—Physical*	Systemic/Multi-Dimensional *Body-Mind-Energy-Spirit*
BEST FOR: Infectious Diseases, Trauma Structural Damage, Organ Failure. Acute Conditions. Lonny J. Brown, Ph.D.	Degenerative, Chronic Stress & Life-style disorders, toxemia, glandular weakness, systemic imbalances.

CHART I.

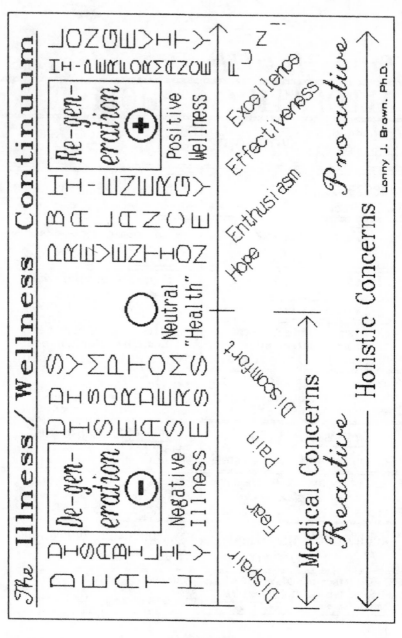

The Illness / Wellness Continuum

Lonny J. Brown. Ph.D.

TRANSCENDENCE

HI-PERFORMANCE

Re-gen-eration (+)

Positive Wellness

HI-ENERGY

BALANCE

PREVENTION

Neutral "Health"

SYMPTOMS

DISORDERS

De-gen-eration (–)

Negative Illness

DISABILITY

DEATH

Fun

Excellence

Effectiveness

Enthusiasm

Hope

Discomfort

Pain

Fear

Despair

← Medical Concerns →
Reactive

Holistic Concerns
Pro-active

CHART 2.

The HOLISTIC SPECTRUM of INTERVENTION

Column headers (left to right): no intervention (prevention · self-healing) | education, counseling & training | Environment | Psycho-Therapies | Energy | Body Therapies | Ingestive Remedies | Pharmacological | Surgical | Terminal Care

---

no intervention / prevention · self-healing · education, counseling & training
- Pattern Analysis – Habit Modification
- HYGIENE
- Motivational Counseling
- Natural Diet / Fasting
- Self-Massage
- Exercise — T'ai Chi
- RELAXATION
- Sports — Biofeedback
- Communication & Assertiveness Training
- Social — Sex & Love
- Inspirational Reading
- Spiritual
- Prayer — Pastoral Counseling
- Visualization
- Meditation
- Autogenic Training
- Yoga
- Breathing Exercises
- Attitudinal Healing
- Lifestyle
- Career & Role Guidance

Environment
- Light & Color
- Hydrotherapy, Whirlpool, Sauna, Sweat Lodge
- Plants & Flowers
- Air Filtration, Ionization
- Sensory Deprivation
- Music
- Nature

Psycho-Therapies
- Analysis
- Transactional
- Humanistic
- Gestalt
- Cognitive
- Motivational
- Expressive
- Transpersonal
- Spiritual
- Past Life Regression
- Guided Imagery
- Medical Astrology
- Primal
- Re-Birthing
- Shamanism
- Placebo
- Hypnosis
- Behavior Modification
- Re-evaluation Co-Counseling

Energy
- Heliotherapy
- Acupuncture, Moxabustion
- Bio-Magnetics
- Therapeutic Touch
- Chakra & Aura Balancing
- Kinesiology
- Polarity
- Radiesthesia, Orgone
- Pranayama
- Reiki

Body Therapies
- Massage, Shiatsu, Acupressure, Reflexology
- Chiropractic
- Yoga
- Osteopathy
- Structural Integration
- Alexander Technique
- Bio-Energetics
- Dance & Movement
- Sex Therapy
- Sports

Ingestive Remedies
- Supplements
- Ortho-Molecular
- Vegetarian
- Juice Fasting
- Macrobiotics
- Herbs
- Therapeutic Foods
- Enzymes
- Homeopathy
- Cell Salts
- Bach Flower Remedies
- Magnetized Water
- Trace Minerals

Pharmacological
- Extracts & Derivatives
- Sedatives, Stimulants
- Chemotherapy
- Psychotropics
- Anti-biotics
- Beta Blockers
- Hormone Replacement
- Narcotics

Surgical
- Transfusion
- Excision
- Organ Replacement
- Bypass

Terminal Care
- Hospice
- Pain Control
- Spiritual Counseling
- Euthanasia

Principles:
- Least Intervention First
- Restore Homeostasis
- Multiple Methods
- "Do No Harm" (Hippocrates)

© Larry J. Brown, Ph.D.

CHART 3.

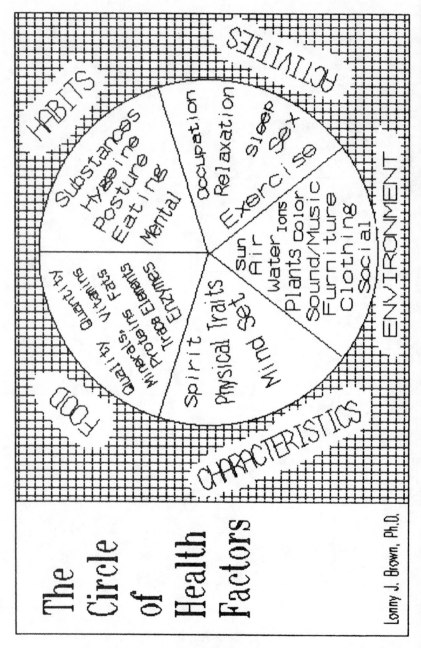

HABITS

ACTIVITIES

ENVIRONMENT

CHARACTERISTICS

FOOD

Substances
Hygiene
Posture
Eating
Mental

Occupation
Relaxation
Sleep
Sex
Exercise

Sun
Air
Water
Ions
Plants
Color
Sound/Music
Furniture
Clothing
Social

Spirit
Physical Traits
Mind Set

Quality
Quantity
Vitamins
Fats
Minerals,
Protein
Trace Elements
Enzymes

The
Circle
of
Health
Factors

Lonny J. Brown, Ph.D.

CHART 4.

Optimum Health Factors

Dimensions	Effective Time Frames				Obstacles
SPIRITUAL	lifetimes / years / months	Inspiration / Guidance Books Teachers Tradition / Path / Ritual Prayer / Meditation Good Karma / Grace Sense of Universal Connection			Ignorance Fear Hatred Doubt Ego Oppression
PHYSICAL	weeks / days	**NUTRITION**	Quality Clean, Fresh, Natural, Whole, Untreated, Local: Vegies Grains Fruit Beans Nuts Seeds Sprouts Herbs, Trace Minerals & Organic Supplements Quantity Systematic Undereating		poor preparation & eating habits junk & fast food poor digestion
		HYGIENE	Internal: clean fresh WATER | Therapeutic Fasting | Colonic Cleansing External: hot water | fresh air | full spectrum SUNLIGHT | skin care natural fibres		poor sanitation & training bacteria pollution
		EXERCISE	Aerobics Sports Play Stretching	Martial Arts Work	laziness tension low energy handicaps
	hours	**RELAXATION**		Sex Massage Stress Reduction Sound Sleep	job stress compulsiveness Addiction Noise
PSYCHOLOGICAL	minutes / seconds	**MENTAL** **EMOTIONAL**	Positive Environment music silence nature space	**MEDITATION**	Cognitive Stress Management Positive Use of Media Mind Training Concentration Visualization & Imagery Creativity / Humor / Curiosity Communication / Supportive Relationships Equanimity LOVE - Rapport Social Inclusion Positive Death Awareness	ignorance oppression depression fear negativity conditioning dullness lust envy hatred

© Lonny J. Brown PhD

CHART 5.

High-Level Wellness

+ Includes Physical Health.
+ Energy. Strength.
+ Safety: Accident Prevention.
+ Peace of Mind: Purpose. Hope. Faith
+ Eqanimity. Balance. Grace.
+ Alertness. Concentration. Curiosity
+ Creativity. Self-Expression.
+ Enthusiasm. Confidence.
+ Love. Sexual Fulfilment.
+ Social & Ecological Awareness
+ Humor. Joy.
+
+
+ -- (Add Your Own Definitions)

CHART 6.

CHAPTER NOTES

I. THE HEALING MIND
1. Locke & Horning-Rohan, 1983.
2. LeShan, 1977.
3. Friedman & Rosenman, 1974.
4. Shapiro, 1970.
5. The Center for Attitudinal Healing. Tiburon, California.
6. "Anatomy of an Illness as Perceived by the Patient," *J. Holistic Health*, Vol. 4, 1979, p. 94.
7. "The Mind as Healer," *Science Digest*, April 1984.
8. Shapiro, p. ii.
9. *Medical Self Care*, No. 23, Winter 1983.
10. Magerey, 1982.
11. *Science Digest*, July 1984.
12. Illich, 1976.
13. LeShan, 1977.
14. Gina Maranto. "Emotions: How they affect your body," *Discover*, Nov. 1984.
    Carroll Nash. "Wishing Spurs Genetic Mutation in Bacteria," *J. Am. S. Psychical Research*, October 1984.
15. "Wholeness, Hippocrates, and Ancient Philosophy," *American Theosophist*, Spring 1984.
16. Ashley Montagu, *Touching—The Human Significance of The Skin*, Harper & Row, 1978.
    See also: Dolores Krieger, Ph.D., R.H., *The Therapeutic Touch*, Prentice Hall, 1979.

II. AUTONOMOUS APPROACHES TO STRESS
1. Cannon, 1939.
2. Margaret Chesney, *SRI Journal*, Dec. 1983, Menlo Park, California.
3. John Leibeskind, *Science 223*: 188-190, 1984.
4. Keller, 1982.
5. Pelletier, 1984.

6. Benson, 1975.
7. Green & Green, 1977.
8. Patel, 1973.
9. Kabat-Zinn, 1984.
10. Soyka, 1977.
11. Rama & Hymes, 1976.
12. Green & Green, 1977.
13. Swami Rama, et. al., 1976.
14. Schwartz, 1978.
15. Green & Green, 1977.
16. Brown, 1978.

III. EATING TO HEAL
1. *Healthline,* Vol. 3, No. 2.
2. McGovern, 1977; Califano, 1979.
3. Health & Longevity Report, June 15, 1984.
4. Christopher, 1976.
5. Airola, 1971; Kulvinskis 1975.

IV. THERAPEUTIC FASTING
1. C.L. Goodrich. "Fasting fosters longevity in rats," *Science News,* Dec. 1, 1979, 116: 375.
   R.H. Weindruch, et.al., "Influence of controlled dietary restriction on immunological function and aging." *Federal Proceedings,* 1979, 38(6): 2007-2016.
2. Metropolitan Life Insurance Co., 1979.
3. Szekely, 1971.
4. Bennett, 1975.
5. Airola, 1972, p. 28-31.
6. V. Young, N. Scrimshaw, "The Psysiology of Starvation," *Scientific American,* Oct. 1971, pp. 14-21.
   J. Am. Med. Ass. October 23/30, 1981, Vol. 246, No. 17, pp. 1878-9.
7. Allan Cott, N.D., and Uri Nickolayev, "Fasting and Schizophrenia." *Schizophrenia,* 1st Quarter, 1971.
   E.J. Drenick, et.al. "Prolonged Starvation Treatment for Severe Obesity," *J. Am. Med. Ass.,* 1964; 167: 100-05.

8. Clark, 1972, p. 367.

9. ibid.

10. *Prevention,* Oct. 1984, p. 61.

11. Airola, 1972; Buchinger, 1972.
    (Dr. Otto Buchinger, Klinik-am Bodensee, 777 Uberlingen, Lake Constance, West Germany. The Buchinger Sanatorium, Bad Pyrmont, West Germany.)

12. Shelton.

13. Ballentine, 1978, pp. 379-380.

14. Airola, 1971, p. 112.

15. ibid. p. 39.

16. The Sacramento Preventive Medicine Clinic. 1816 Tribute Rd., Sacramento, CA 95815. (916) 925-7811.

17. Airola, Paavo, N.D., Ph.D., 1971, p. 112.

18. ibid. p. 22-23.

19. Cahill, G.F. Jr., Herrera M.G., Morgan A.P., et.al. "Hormone-fuel interrelationships during fasting." *J. Clin. Investigation.* 45: 1751-1769, 1966.
    Cahill G.F. Jr., Owen O.E., Morgan A.P., "The Consumption of fuels during prolonged starvation." *Advances in Enzyme Regulation.* 6: 143-150. 1968.
    Hundler, R.G., et. al. "Epinephrine-stimulated glucose production is not diminished by starvation: evidence for an effect on gluconeogenesis." *J. Clin. Endoc. Metab.* 1984, June; 58 (6): 1014-1021.

20. Airola, Paavo, Ph.D., N.D., 1971, p. 124.

21. Dr. Steven Cordas, Clinical Ecology Unit, Northeast Community Hospital. Bedford, TX 76022.

22. Shelton, Herbert M., 1978, p. 165.

23. Kerndt, P.R., M.D.; Naughton, J.L., M.D.; Driscoll, .C.E., M.D.; & Loxterkamp, D.S. M.D. "Fasting: The History, Pathophysiology and Complications." *Western J. of Med.,* Nov. 1982, 134:5, p. 394.

24. Kerndt, et.al. op. cit., p. 380.

V. THE SPIRIT OF HEALING

1. *The American Theosophist.* Spring, 1984.

2. *REVISION*, Spring 1984, Vol. 7, No. 1.
3. Green & Green, 1977.
4. *Assoc. Humanistic Psycho. Newsletter*, Sept. 1979.
5. *ECAP*, 2 Church St. South, New Haven, CT 06519.
6. ibid.
7. From the ECAP brochure.

VI. IN YOGA AS IN LIFE
1. Shealy 1976; Kabat-Zinn, 1984. *Dr. Kabat-Zinn has been teaching Buddhist mindfullness meditation and Yoga techniques at the Chronic Pain Control program at University of Massachusetts Hospital.*

VII. CORE RELAXATION
1. Wilhelm Reich, 1973.

VIII. THE PICTURE OF HEALTH : VISUALIZATION
1. *Science Digest*, August 1984.
2. OMM Corp., P.O. Box 767, Deerfield, IL 60015.
3. Achterberg & Lawliss, 1980.
4. Green & Green, 1977.
5. E.H. Shattock, 1982.

X. ANNE : A PERSONAL ACCOUNT
1. See *The Healing Power of Laughter & Play: Uses of Humor in the Healing Arts* (The Second Annual Conference, 1983. The Institute for the Advancement of Human Behavior. Stanford, California, w/Interface/AHMA.)
2. Dr. Watson Reid, McLean Hospital, Belmont, MA.

BIBLIOGRAPHY

Acciardo, Marcia. 1978. *Light Eating For Survival.* OmanGod Press, Woodstock Valley, CT.

Achterberg, Jeanne, Ph.D. 1985. *"Imagery of Healing—Shamanism & Modern Medicine.* Shambhala/New Science Library, Boston & London.

_____. 1976. O. Carl Simonton, M.D., and Stephanie Matthews-Simonton. 1976. *Stress, Psychological Factors and Cancer.* Cancer Counseling & Research Center, Fort Worth, TX.

_____, & G. Frank Lawliss. 1980. *Bridges of the BodyMind—Behavioral Approaches to Health Care.* Institute for Personality and Ability Testing, Inc. Champaign, IL.

Airola, Paavo, Ph.D., N.D. 1968. *There Is A Cure For Arthritis.* Parker Publishing Co., West Nyack, NY.

_____. 1972. *Cancer: The Total Approach.* Health Plus, Phoenix, AZ.

_____. 1971. *Are You Confused?* Health Plus, Phoenix, AZ.

_____. 1974. *How To Get Well.* Health Plus, Phoenix, AZ.

_____. 1971. *How To Keep Slim, Healthy & Young With Juice Fasting.* Health Plus, Phoenix, AZ.

_____. 1972. *Health Secrets From Europe.* Arco Publishing Co., New York.

Ajaya, Swami, ed. 1976. *Meditational Therapy.* Himalayan International Institute, Honesdale, PA.

Anderson, Bob. 1980. *Stretching.* Shelter Publishing, Bolinas, California.

Ardell, Donald B. 1977. *High Level Wellness.* Rodale Press, Emmaus, Pennsylvania.

Assagioli, Roberto, 1976. *Psychosynthesis.* Penguin, New York.

Aurobindo, Sri, and The Mother. n.d. *On Illness.* The Sri Aurobindo Society, Pondicherry, India.

Ballentine, Rudolph M.D., Swami Ajaya, Phillip Nurernberger, PhD., Charles Bates, Jagdish Dave, Ph.D., 1979. *Therapeutic Value of Yoga.* Himalayan International Institute, Honesdale, Pennsylvania.

Bates, W.H., M.D. 1973. *Better Eyesight Without Glasses.* Pyramid, New York.

Bennett, John G. 1975. *Long Pilgrimage—The Life & Teachings of the Shiva Puri Baba.* Rainbow Bridge, San Francisco.

Benson, Herbert, M.D. 1979. *The Mind/Body Effect.* Simon & Shuster, New York.

————. 1975. *The Relaxation Response.* Avon, New York.

————. 1984. *Beyond the Relaxation Response.* Times Books, New York.

————. 1987. *Your Maximum Mind.* Random House, NY.

Berkeley Holistic Health Center. 1986. *The Holistic Health Handbook.* And/Or Book Conspiracy, Berkeley, California.

Borassenko, Joan. 1987. *Minding the Body, Mending the Mind.*

Brena, Steven F., M.D. 1972. *Yoga and Medicine.* Penguin Books, New York.

Bricklin, Steven F., M.D. *The Practical Encyclopedia of Natural Healing*

Brown, Barbara. 1974. *New Mind, New Body.* Bantam, New York.

————. 1978. *Stress and the Art of Biofeedback.* Bantam, New York.

————. 1984. *Between Health and Illness.* Houghton Mifflin, Boston.

Brown, Lonny J., Ph.D. 1979. *Beginner's Meditation: Questions & Answers.* Greenfield, NH 03047.

Bry, Adelaide. 1978. *Directing the Movies of Your Mind.* Harper & Row, New York.

Buchinger, Otto H.F. 1972. *Everything You Want to Know About Fasting.* Pyramid Books, New York.

Byron, Thomas (trans.) 1976. *The Dhammapada.* Alfred A. Knopf, New York.

Califano, Joseph. 1979. *Healthy People: The United States Surgeon General's Report on Health Promotion and Disease.*

Cannon, Walter B. 1939. *The Wisdom of the Body.* 2nd ed. Worton, New York.

Cancer Counseling and Research Center. n.d. *Cancer Self-Help Education.* Health Education Programs, Saratoga, California.

Carlson, Rick, J., ed. 1975. *The Frontiers Science and Medicine,* Henry Regnery Co., Chicago.

Carrington, Patricia, Ph.D. 1978. *Freedom in Meditation.* Anchor/Doubleday, New York.

_____. 1984. *Releasing.* William Morrow, New York.

Challoner, H.K. 1976. *The Path of Healing.* Quest/Theosophical, Wheaton, Illinois.

Chopra, Deepak, M.D. 1987. *Creating Health—Beyond Prevention, Toward Perfection.* Houghton Mifflin, Boston.

Christopher, John R. 1976. *School of Natural Healing.* Dr. John Christopher Pub., Provo, Utah.

Clark, Linda. 1965. *Get Well Naturally.* ARC Books, New York.

Conze, Edward. 1956. *Buddhist Meditation.* Harper & Row, New York.

Cook, Ivan. 1976. *Healing By The Spirit.* The White Eagle Publishing Trust, Hampshire, England.

Cousins, Norman. 1979. *Anatomy of An Illness (as Perceived by the Patient).* W.W. Norton & Co., New York.

_____. 1983. *The Healing Heart—Antidotes to Panic & Helplessness.* W.W. Norton & Co., New York.

Dass, Ram. 1978. *Journey of Awakening: A Meditator's Guidebook.* Bantam, New York.

Davis, Adelle, 1970. *Let's Eat Right To Keep Fit.* American Library, Bergenfield, New Jersey.

Davis, Martha, Ph.D., Matthew McKay, Ph.D. & Elizabeth Robbins Eshelman. 1980. *The Relaxation & Stress Reduction Workbook.* New Harbinger Publ., Richmond, California.

Dharma-Sara. 1976. *Between Pleasure & Pain.* Dharma-Sara Pub., Sumas, Washington.

_____, Matthew McKay, Ph.D., & Patrick Fanning. 1981. *Thoughts & Feelings—The Art of Cognitive Stress Intervention.* New Harbinger Publ., Richmond, California.

Dossey, Larry, M.D. 1984. *Beyond Illness—Discovering the Experience of Health.* Shambhala/New Science Library, Boulder, CO, & London.

Dychtwald, Ken. 1977. *Bodymind.* Harcourt-Brace, New York.

Eccles, John C. 1973. *The Understanding of the Brain.* McGraw-Hill, 1973.

Edmunds, H. Tudor, ed. 1976. *Some Unrecognized Factors in Medicine.* Quest/Theosophical Pub., Wheaton, Illinois.

Fadiman, James, & Robert Frager, 1976. *Personality & Personal Growth.* Harper & Row, New York.

Foundation for Inner Peace. 1975. *A Course In Miracles.* F.I.P, Washington, D.C.

Friedman, Meyer, M.D. & Ray H. Sosenman, M.D. 1975. *Type "A" Behavior and Your Heart.* Fawcett Publishers, Greenwich, Connecticut.

Funderburk, James, Ph.D. 1977. *Science Studies Yoga.* Himalayan International Institute, Honesdale, Pennsylvania.

Gandhi, M.K. 1965. *The Health Guide.* The Crossing Press, Trumansburg, New York.

Gardner, Adelaide, 1968. *Meditation, A Practical Study.* Quest, Wheaton, Illinois.

Girdano, Daniel A., Ph.D. & George S. Everly, Jr., Ph.D. 1979. *Controlling Stress and Tension.* Prentice-Hall, Englewood Cliffs, New Jersey.

Goldstein, Joseph. 1976. *The Experience of Insight.* Unity, Santa Cruz, California.

Goleman, Daniel. 1977. *Varieties of the Meditative Experience.* Dutton, New York.

Gordon, Jafee, & Bresler, n.d. *Mind, Body & Health—Toward an Integral Medicine.* Human Science Press.

Green, Elmer and Alyce. 1977. *Beyond Biofeedback.* Dell, NY.

Hanh, Thich Nhat. 1975. *The Miracle of Being Awake.* Fellowship Books, Nyak, New York.

Hay, Louise. 1984. *You Can Heal Your Life.* Hay House, Santa Monica, California.

Halifax, Joan, 1979. *Shamanic Voices: A Survey of Visionary Narratives.* Dutton, New York.

Heline, Corrinne. 1976. *Healing and Regeneration Through Color.* New Age Press, Los Angeles.

Hirai, Tomio. 1975. *Zen Meditation Therapy.* Japan Publications Trading Co., Elmsford, New York.

Hodgkinson, Neville. 1986. *Will To Be Well—The Real Alternative Medicine.* Samual Weiser, York Beach, Maine.

Hulke, Malcolm, ed. 1979. *The Encyclopedia of Alternative Medicine and Self-Help.*

Hunter, Beatrice Trum. 1979. *The Mirage of Safety: Food Additives & Federal Policy.* Charles Scribner's Sons, New York.

Hurd, Frank J., D.C. 1968. *Ten Talents—A Good Cook.* Box 86A, Rt. 1, Chisholm, MN 55719.

Hutschnecker, A.A. 1953. *The Will To Live.* Thomas Y. Crowel Co., New York.

Illich, Ivan. 1976. *Medical Nemisis: The Expropriation of Health.* Bantam, New York.

Iyengar, B.K.S. 1966. *Light On Yoga.* Schocken, New York.

Jackson, M., & T. Teague. 1975. *The Handbook of Alternatives to Chemical Medicine.* Lawton Teague.

Jacobson, Edmund. 1974. *Progressive Relaxation.* University of Chicago Press, Chicago.

Jaffe, Dennis T., Ph.D. 1980. *Healing From Within.* Alfred A. Knopf, New York.

Jensen, Bernard, D.C. n.d. *Tissue Cleansing Through Bowel Management.* Hidden Valley Health Ranch, Rt. 1 Box 52, Escondido, CA 92025.

_____. *A New Lifestyle for Health & Happiness—A Compilation of Wholistic Healing Wisdom.*

_____. *Food Healing for Man.*

Jy, Brugh. 1978. *Joy's Way—A Map for the Transformational Journey.* Los Angeles: J.P. Tarcher, Inc. 1978.

Keller, Kathleen Lahr. 1982. *Burnout in Baccalaureate Nursing Students as It Relates to Self-Actualization and Coping Methods* (Ph.D. Diss.) University of Southern California.

Kelley, Dr. Wm. Donald. 1974. *One Answer to Cancer.* International Association of Cancer Victims & Friends, Beverly Hills, California.

Kennett, Roshi Jiyu. 1977. *How to Grow a Lotus Blossom.* Shasta Abbey, Mt. Shasta, California.

Khan, Sufi Inayat. 1961. *The Development of Spiritual Healing.* Sufi Publications, Geneva.

Kloss, Jethro. 1972. *Back to Eden.* Lifeline Books, Riverside, California.

Krieger, Dolores. 1981. *Foundations for Holistic Health Nursing Practices—the Renaissance Nurse.* J.B Lippincott Co., Philadelphia, Penn.

Kulvinskas, Viktoras. 1975. *Survival Into The 21st Century.* OmanGod Press, Wethersfield, Connecticut.

Lappe, Frances Moore. 1971. *Diet for A Small Planet.* Ballantine, New York.

LeShan, Lawrence. 1974. *How To Meditate.* Bantam, New York.

_____. 1977. *Your Can Fight For Your Life—Emotional Factors in the Treatment of Cancer.* M. Evans & Co., New York.

Levine, Stephen. 1979. *A Gradual Awakening.* Anchor, Garden City, New York.

Locke, Dr. Steven. *Mind and Immunity: Behavioral Immunology.* New York Institute for the Advancement of Health. 16 E. 53 St., New York, NY 10022.

Luthe, W. 1969. *Autogenic Therapy.* Grune & Stratton, New York.

Macdonald-Bayne. 1940. *Heal Yourself.* Lowe and Brydone, Ltd., Norfolk, England.

Mae, Eydie. 1975. *How I Conquered Cancer Naturally.* Production House, San Diego.

Mandell, Marshall, M.D. n.d. *Lifetime Arthritis Relief System.* G. Sanders Books, Hurst, Texas.

Mangalo, Bhikkhu. 1978. *The Practice of Recollection—A Guide to Buddhist Meditation.* Prajna Press, Boulder, Colorado.

Mason, L. John. Ph.D. 1980. *Guide to Stress Reduction.* Peace Press, Inc., Culver City, California.

Master, Robert, & Jean Houston. 1978. *Listening to the Body.* Delacort, Boston.

McGovern, George, 1977. *Dietary Goals for the United States.* U.S. Government Printing Office.

McKay, Matthew, Ph.D., Martha Davis, Ph.D. & Patrick Fanning. 1981. *Thoughts & Feelings. The Art of Cognitive Stress Intervention.* New Harbinger Publications, Richmond, California.

Meek, George W. 1977. *Healers and the Healing Process.* Quest/ Theosophical Press, Wheaton, Illinois.

Moss, Richard M.D. 1981. *The I That Is We—Awakening to Higher Energies Through Unconditional Love.* Celestial Arts, Millbrae, California.

Naranjo, Claudio, & Robert E. Ornstein, 1973. *On the Psychology of Meditation.* Viking Press, New York.

Ott, John N. 1976. *Health and Light.* Simon & Shuster, New York.

Oyle, Irving. M.D. 1979. *The New American Medicine Show.* Unity Press, Santa Cruz.

_____. 1976. *Magic, Mysticism, and Modern Medicine.* Celestial Arts, Millbrae, California.

_____. 1976. *Time, Space and the Mind.* Celestial Arts, Millbrae, California.

Padus, Emrika. 1986. *The Complete Guide to Your Emotions & Your Health—New Dimensions in Mind/Body Healing.* Rodale Press, Emmaus, Penn.

Parampanthi, Swami. 1974. *Creative Self-Transformation Through Meditation.* Astara, Los Angeles.

Pelletier, Kenneth R. 1977. *Mind As Healer, Mind As Slayer.* Dell, New York.

_____. 1978. *Toward A Science of Consciousness.* Dell, New York.

_____. 1980. *Holistic Medicine. From Stress to Optimum Health.* Dell, New York.

_____. 1981. *Longevity—Fullfilling Our Biological Potential.* Delecorte & Delta, New York.

_____. 1984. *Healthy People in Unhealthy Places—Stress & Fitness At Work.* Delecorte & Delta, New York.

Popenoe, Chris. 1977. *Wellness.* Yes! Books, Washington, D.C.

Porter, Garrett, & Patricia A. Norris, Ph.D. 1986. *Why Me!—Harnessing The Healing Power of the Human Spirit.* Stillpoint Press, Walpole, New Hampshire.

Prabhavananda, Swami, & Christopher Isherwood. 1969. *How To Know God: The Yoga Aphorisms of Patanjali.* Signet, New York.

Progoff, Dr. Ira. 1971. *The Well and the Cathredral.* Dialogue House, New York.

_____. 1972. *The White Robed Monk*. Dialogue House, New York.

_____. 1975. *At A Journal Workshop*. Dialogue House, New York.

Rama, Swami, Rudolph Ballentine, M.D. & Swami Ajaya (Allan Weinstock, Ph.D.) 1976. *Yoga and Psychotherapy—The Evolution of Consciousness*. Himalayan Institute, Glenview, Illinois.

_____, Rudolph Ballenine, M.D., & Alan Hymes, M.D. n.d., *Science of Breath—A Practical Guide*. Himalayan Publishers, Honesdale, Penn.

Ramacharaka, Yogi. 1937. *The Science of Psychic Healing*. Yogi Publications Society, Chicago.

Reich, Wilhelm. 1973. *The Cancer Biopathy*. Farrar, Straus & Giroux, 1973.

Rolfe, Lionel, and Nigey Lennon. 1983. *The Heal Yourself Home Handbook of Unusual Remedies*. Parker Publishing, West Nyak, New York.

Ross, Shirley. 1976. *Fasting: The Super Diet*. Ballantine, New York.

Ryan, Regina Sara, & John W. Travis, M.D. 1981. *The Wellness Workbook*, Ten Speed Press, Berkeley.

Sammuels, Michael, and Hal Bennett. 1973. *The Well Body Book*. Random House/Bookworks, New York.

Samuels, Mike, M.D. & Nancy Samuels. 1975. *Seeing With the Mind's Eye—The History, Techniques & Uses of Visualization*. Random House/Bookworks, New York/Berkeley.

Schiffman, M. 1967. *Gestalt Self-Therapy*. Self-Therapy Press, Menlo Park, California.

Schwartz, Gary, E., Ph.D. n.d. *Relaxation, Meditation & Stress Management*. BMA Audio Cassette Publ. NY 10003. (A taped lecture.)

Schwarz, Jack. 1978. *Voluntary Controls*. E.P. Dutton, New York.

Sehnert, Keith W., M.D. 1975. *How To Be Your Own Doctor (Sometimes)*. Grosset and Dunlap, New York.

Selye, Hans. 1976. *The Stress of Life*. McGraw Hill, New York.

_____. 1974. *Stress Without Distress.* New Age Foods, Boulder, Colorado.

Shapiro, Arthur K. 1979. *A Contribution to the History of the Placebo Effect.* Elmcrest Psychiatric Institute, Portland, Connecticut.

Shattock, E.H. 1982. *A Manual of Self-Healing.* Destiny Books, New York.

Shealy, C. Norman, & Arthur S. Freese. 1975. *Occult Medicine Can Save Your Life.* Dial, New York.

_____. 1977. *90 Days to Self-Health.* Dial, New York.

_____. 1976. *The Pain Game.* Celestial Arts, Millbrae, CA.

_____, & Caroline Myss, M.A. 1987. *The Creation of Health—The Merger of Traditional Medical Diagnosis With Clairvoyant Insight.* Stillpoint, Walpole, New Hampshire.

Sheikh, Anees, A., Ed. 1984. *Imagination and Healing—Imagery and Human Development.* Vol. 1. Baywood Publishing, Farmingdale, New York.

Sheldrake, Rupert. 1982. *A New Science of Life—The Hypothesis of Formative Causation.* J.P. Tarcher, Los Angeles.

Shelton, Herbert M. 1964. *Fasting Can Save Your Life.* Natural Hygiene Press, Chicago.

Siegal, Bernie S., M.D. 1986. *Love, Medicine, & Miracles—Lessons Learned About Self-Healing from a Surgeon's Experience With Exceptional Patients.* Harper & Row, New York.

Simeons, A.J.W. 1961. *Man's Presumptuous Brain.* Dutton, New York.

Simonton, O. Carl, Stephanie Matthew-Simonton, & Rames L. Creighton. 1981. *Getting Well Again.* Bantam, New York.

Soyka, Fred. 1977. *The Ion Effect—How Air Electricity Rules Your Life & Health.* Dutton, New York.

Stone, Randolph. *Health Building—The Conscious Art of Living Well.* CRCS Publishers, Reno. n.d.

Suzuki, Shunryu. 1970. *Zen Mind, Beginner's Mind.* Weatherhill, New York.

Szekely, Edmund Bordeaux, ed. & trans. 1971. *The Essene Gospel of Peace.* Academy of Creative Living, San Diego.

_____. 1970. *The Essene Science of Life.*

_____. 1975. *The Essene Science of Fasting.*

_____. 1978. *The Book of Vitamins.*

_____. 1978. *The Book of Minerals.*

Tarthang Tulku, Ed. 1977. *Calm & Clear.* Dharma, Emeryville, California.

Theosophical Research Centre. 1958. *The Mystery of Healing.* Quest/Theosophical Pub., Wheaton, Illinois.

Thera, Nyanaponika. 1962. *The Heart of Recollection—A Guide to Buddhist Meditation.* Weiser, New York.

Tilden, J.H., M.D. n.d. *Toxemia Explained.* Health Research, Mokelumne Hill, California.

Travis, J. 1977. *Wellness Workbook.* Wellness Resource Center, Mill Valley, California.

Trungpa, Chogyam. 1976. *The Myth of Freedom.* Shambhala, Berkeley.

Vaughan, Frances E. Ph.D. 1979. *Awakening Intuition.* Anchor, New York.

Villoldo, Alberto, & Stanley Kripper. 1966. *Realms of Healing.* Celestial Arts.

Vishnudevananda, Swami. 1960. *The Complete Illustrated Book of Yoga.* Simon & Shuster, New York.

Walker, Evan Harris. 1970. "Consciousness and Quantum Theory" *Psychic Exploration: A Challenge for Science.* J. White, ed. New York: G.P. Putnam's Sons, 1970.

Ward, Milton. 1977. *The Brilliant Function of Pain.* Optimus Books, New York.

Watts, Alan. 1974. *Meditation: How To Do It.* Pyramid, New York.

Weil, Andrew, 1984. *Health and Healing.* Houghton Mifflin, Boston.

Welwood, John, Ed. 1983. *Awakening the Heart—East/West Approaches to Psychotherapy & the Healing Relationships.* Shambhala, Boulder, Colorado.

Whole Health Institute. n.d. *Health in the Colon.* Health Institute, Leominster, Mass.

Winters, Jason. 1982. *Killing Cancer.* M & R Publishers, Las Vegas.

Woods, Nancy Fugate. 1979. *Human Sexuality in Health and Illness.* 2nd Ed. C.V. Mosby Co., St. Louis.

Yogananda, Paramahansa. 1959. *Autobiography of a Yogi.* Self Realization Fellowship, Los Angeles.

Young, Lawrence, M.D. ed. 1980. *Reports of the National Clearinghouse for Meditation Relaxation and Related Therapies.* P.O. Box 3184. New York 10008.

ARTICLES:

Borysenki, Joan. "Psychoneuroimmunology: Behavioral Factors and the Immune Response," *REVISION,* Spring 1984. (P.O. Box 316, Cambridge, MA 02238.)

Chesney, Margaret. "On Personality Type/Job Mismatching & Stress," *SRI Journal.* Dec. 1983. Menlo Park. CA.

Clark, Carolyn Chambers. "Using Guided Imagery to Reduce Blood Pressure," 1983. *The Wellness Newsletter.* July/ August.

Cohen, David. 1975. "Magnetic Fields of the Human Body," *Physics Today,* August 1975. 34-43.

Hammer, Signe. 1984. "The Mind As Healer," *Science Digest.* April.

Ingrasci, Rick, M.D. 1979. "The Universe is a Placebo," *New Age Journal.* May.

Kabat-Zinn, Jon. 1982. "An Outpatient Program in Behavioral Medicine For Chronic Pain Patients Based on the Practice of Mindfulness Meditation: Theoretical Considerations & Preliminary Results," *General Hospital Psychiatry.* 4: -47.

_____. "Coping With Chronic Pain: An Interview With Jon Kabat-Zinn," *REVISION Journal.* Vol. 7 No. 1: Consciousness & Healing: Shifting Currents in Contemporary Medicine.

Levy, Sandra M. 1984. "Emotions and the Progression of Cancer: A Review," *Advances, Journal of the Institute for the Advancement of Health,* Vol. 1, No. 1, Winter.

_____. "Host Differences in Neoplastic Risk: Behavioral and Social Contributors to Disease," *Health Psychology,* 2:21.44. 1983.

Liebeskind, Lewis, Shavit, Terman, & Melnechuk. 1983. "Our Natural Capacities for Pain Suppression," *Advances, Journal of the Institute for the Advancement of Health.* Vol. 1, November.

MacNutt, Francis, Ph.D. 1984. "What I Have Learned in Praying for Healing," *Journal of Holistic Health,* Vol. 9, Mandala, Delmar, CA.

Magarey, C. 1982. "Holistic Cancer Therapy," *Journal of Psychological Research.* 27: 18184.

O'Regan, Brendan, & Rick J. Carlson. 1979. "Defining Health: The State of the Art," *Holistic Health Review.* Winter.

Patel, C.H. 1973. "Yoga & Biofeedback in the Management of Hypertension," *The Lancet,* November, pp. 1053-1055.

Vaughan, Frances, Ph.D. 1983. "Chakra Symbolism—A Psychological Commentary" *The American Theosophist,* Fall, Wheaton, Illinois.

Wingerson, L "Training the Mind to Heal," *Discover.* May 1982. 80-85.

Winstock. C. "Recent Progress in Cancer Psychobiology & Psychiatry," *Journal of the American Society for Psychosomatic Dental Medicine,* 1977; 24:4-14.

"Psychosocial Determinants of Immunologically Mediated Diseases" (Conference Report), *Advances: Journal of the Institute for the Advancement of Health,* Vol. 1, No. 1, Winter 1984.

"Shamans and Endorphins," *Ethos.* Vol. 10, No. 4, Winter 1982.

"Self-Healing," *New Age Journal,* May 1979.

"Recent Progress in Cancer Psychobiology and Psychiatry," *Journal of the American Society for Psychosomatic Dental Medicine.* 1977; 24:4-14.

"How Doctors Cause Disease," *Medical Self-Care.* No. 23, Winter 1983.

"Emotions: How They Affect Your Body," *Discover.* November 1984.